Reversing Memory Loss

Reversing Memory Loss

Proven Methods for Regaining, Strengthening, and Preserving Your Memory

Vernon H. Mark, M.D., F.A.C.S.
with Jeffrey P. Mark, M.Sc.

Houghton Mifflin Company   *Boston New York London   1992*

For information about permission to reproduce selections from this book, write to Permissions, Houghton Mifflin Company, 215 Park Avenue South, New York, New York 10003.

Library of Congress Cataloging-in-Publication Data
Mark, Vernon H., date.
  Reversing memory loss : proven methods for regaining, strengthening, and preserving your memory / Vernon H. Mark with Jeffrey P. Mark.
      p.   cm.
  Includes bibliographical references (p.) and index.
  ISBN 0-395-55220-6
  1. Memory disorders — Prevention.   2. Memory disorders in old age — Prevention.   3. Memory.   I. Mark, J. Paul.   II. Title.
RC394.M46M37   1992   91-36598
616.8'4 — dc20   CIP

Printed in the United States of America

AGM 10 9 8 7 6 5 4 3 2 1

The information presented in case histories and stories in *Reversing Memory Loss* is medically accurate. However, all names, places, and characteristics that could identify specific individuals have been changed to protect privacy. Some case histories contain elements from more than one patient. Any resemblance to persons living or dead is coincidental.

Before you start the regimens presented in this book, consult your own physician to make sure that they are suitable for you.

None of the information presented here is intended to substitute for medical advice. If you have any problems or questions related to your own health and fitness, you should direct them to your physician.

For Alexandra

———

For "Paws"

Acknowledgments

MANY OF THE SAME individuals who helped in the preparation of our previous book, *Brain Power*, were also of great assistance on this book. Again, my co-author, Jeffrey Mark, and I would especially like to thank Ruth Hapgood of Houghton Mifflin, whose enthusiasm and dedication have never wavered. We were truly blessed to have such a talented and knowledgeable editor. Becky Saikia-Wilson, supervisor of manuscript editing, and Rachel Parks, manuscript editor, worked with us on *Brain Power* and again on this book. In both cases their work was exemplary. Mab Gray of Houghton Mifflin's publicity department spent long hours helping us with promotion, and we would like to acknowledge her tireless efforts. Sue Tecce of Houghton Mifflin's editorial department was very helpful throughout the writing, editing, and production stages. We are extremely happy to have Flip Brophy of Sterling Lord Literistic represent us, and we thank her for her timely advice and assistance.

I am pleased to have the chance to thank my friend, partner, and colleague, Dr. Thomas D. Sabin. Although neither of us will admit to being that old, our collaboration has now spanned more than twenty-five years. I feel very fortunate to have worked with Tom, one of the top neurologists in the world, for so long.

As always, I am grateful for the talents of Joyce Sabin of Sabin & Mark, who has guided our enterprise through difficult times. I'd also like to thank Elec Toth and Mary Grace Neal, who have helped Sabin & Mark (both the company and the doctors themselves) in so many ways.

Dr. Jonathan Lieff has been a good friend and trusted associate for a number of years, and I am proud that he has written the foreword to this book.

All errors in fact or judgment are exclusively my own.

VERNON H. MARK, M.D., F.A.C.S.

Contents

Foreword

In my experience as a geriatric psychiatrist, memory loss is the reason most people in nursing homes are unable to live independently. Whether that loss is the result of depression, metabolic disturbance, malnutrition, Alzheimer's disease, multi-infarct dementia, stroke, tumor, or any of a variety of major brain injuries or diseases, the result is the same. Without the ability to remember, without the storehouse of memories that allow us to carry out routine functions of daily living, we lose our independence.

America is undeniably getting older. Within the next twenty years many in the "baby boom" generation of the late 1940s and early 1950s will be at the age where they may need to enter nursing homes. But America's nursing homes are already overcrowded, and many are unable to provide the complex of treatment needed for the many different types of patients. Is the solution to build more nursing homes? The answer is really a new vision of care for the elderly and new ways of keeping elderly people out of nursing homes as long as possible. This is the promise of the broader view expressed in *Reversing Memory Loss*.

My initial exposure to Dr. Mark's work came more than twelve years ago when he consulted with several patients that I was treating in nursing homes. Since then I have observed his comprehensive evaluations of many patients. Dr. Mark has had extensive experience in treating the elderly and has studied the issues of nursing home care in great detail. At his Center for Memory Impairment and Neurobehavioral Disorders (CMIND), he coordinated the work of a multidisciplinary team of professionals providing the types of treatment described in this book.

Dr. Mark has always impressed me with his great depth of knowledge about medicine and about his patients. He has the qualities that I respect most in a physician, that is, the ability to concentrate on, and creatively study, all of a patient's relevant symptoms; the vision to pay special attention to the way these many details impinge upon a patient's life; and the energy to care enough about his patients to help them change. In evaluating the brain, and especially the complex disorders of memory, this type of concern is vital.

We are truly at a crossroads in medicine and history. The explosion of information, a result of billions of dollars spent on research, will soon pay enormous dividends. Soon various forms of heart disease and cancer may be entirely curable. As important as those problems are, we must never lose sight of the fact that the brain is ultimately what controls life, and it is our ability to remember that permits us to thrive. *Reversing Memory Loss* prods us to keep medical progress in perspective. What use is a perfectly healthy heart if the brain is unable to remember how to cross a street without being hit by a car?

Alexander Smith once wrote, "A man's real possession is his memory. In nothing else is he rich, in nothing else is he poor." *Reversing Memory Loss* will help everyone who reads it to protect their most vital possession. It contains the collected wisdom of hundreds of medical experts and the most up-to-the-minute information on what each of us can do to reverse the processes that cause memory loss.

FOREWORD

I encourage everyone, young and old, to take this book to
heart and to make the changes that can lead to a healthier,
happier, and more productive life.

JONATHAN D. LIEFF, M.D.
President, American Association for Geriatric Psychiatry (1990–
1991)
Fellow, American Psychiatric Association
Associate Clinical Professor of Psychiatry, Boston University
Medical School
Diplomate of the American Board of Psychiatry and Neurology,
with Added Qualification in Geriatric Psychiatry
Chief of Psychiatry, Hahnemann Hospital and American Geriatric
Service

Take Charge of Your Life

ARE YOU HAVING TROUBLE remembering things? Do the names of people you've met a dozen times suddenly escape you? Do you ever come into a room to perform a specific task and forget what you wanted to do? You're not alone. Many millions of people share your complaints, and hundreds of thousands regularly worry that they're losing their memories (the first sign, they think, that they're losing their minds), to the point that they seek professional medical advice.

Let me reassure you that the overwhelming majority of these complaints are not associated with Alzheimer's disease or irreversible memory loss. Even if you feel that your memory loss persists, you should not become fearful that the meaningful period of your life has suddenly ended. What you may need to do is undergo medical testing to find out what's wrong, then have the underlying problem corrected. The important thing for you to keep in mind is that many kinds of memory loss can be easily diagnosed and treated.

As you'll learn, there are many different kinds of memory, all of which are controlled by the brain, and all of which are important. However, one kind of memory is essential. It is at the center or core of memory; indeed, it is at the core of your being, representing the essential you, your personality, your

1

feelings. It is called vital memory, and all other forms of memory are rooted in this function.

Sometimes it's difficult to understand how crucial vital memory is in our lives until we see what happens when it's destroyed. In early 1990, a woman testified before Congress about a weight-loss program her forty-five-year-old husband had enrolled in less than a year before. He had been about thirty pounds overweight, and the weight-loss clinic put him on a liquid diet that did, in fact, cause him to shed his unwanted pounds. But one day when the man was out jogging he suddenly had a stroke, the result of the kind of diet he was on, which left him in a coma. Even though he was at first paralyzed and unable to speak, intensive therapy over a period of several months improved his speech and arm and leg functions to the point that he was almost normal. He was left, however, with one critical deficiency: he had lost his vital memory. He had lost all memory of prior events, including who he was, who his wife and children were, and what had been his hopes and dreams for the future.

The man's wife was justifiably bitter. Without his vital memory, she explained, he looked the same, spoke in the same way, and did many things as he had before. Yet he was only a shadow of his former self — a Hollywood facade with no underlying structure. When his vital memory had gone, all the things that made him a unique individual also disappeared. His body was rehabilitated; his mind was not.

Such selective loss of vital memory following a stroke is very uncommon. What this man's experience illustrates, however, is not just that a stroke can be tremendously debilitating, but that his stroke could have been prevented with proper precautions. Moreover, other kinds of memory loss, even those associated with some strokes, can be reversed.

This book is about memory, but it is unlike others that address the topic. Books such as *Thirty Days to a Better Memory, Business Success Through Memory,* and *New Secrets of Im-*

proving Your Memory — and literally hundreds of others of the same variety — are clearly helpful to those of us who want to improve intellectual capacity. But such improvements, nice as they are, are trivial compared to preserving vital memory and reversing the loss of our selves.

Vital memory is one of the most basic and necessary functions of our brains. The cartoonist Gary Larson captured the essence of vital memory in one of his "Far Side" cartoons. An elderly man with a stubble of whiskers wakes up in the morning. Beside the man's bed is a large poster with block letters reminding him, PUT YOUR PANTS ON BEFORE THE SHOES! When you wake up each morning, do you know where you are, who you are, and what the date is? Do you remember what happened the day before, and how it affected you? Do you have a general idea of how you fit into your surroundings? Most important, do you know what your plans and expectations for the immediate future are — the rest of the morning, the afternoon, the evening, tomorrow?

If you retain your vital memory, you will continue to be in charge of your own life. If you don't, life will not have much meaning for you. You become an object rather than a person, someone to be taken care of. The less vital memory you have, the more your individual freedom is compromised. As long as you retain your vital memory you are a going concern, no matter how old you are. Even if some of your memory resources are reduced, or if your visual or hearing memories are diminished, you'll still be able to take care of yourself.

The reason I stress vital memory as the core of your memory function is to give you some perspective on your memory complaints. The more superficial aspects of memory may be deficient from time to time in all of us — you and me included. And when you have problems such as difficulty in recalling a name, forgetting the context of a conversation, having an idea pop into your head and leave just as quickly, you should not be unduly alarmed as long as your vital memory is intact.

This book touches on a number of aspects of memory and memory loss, but the subject of vital memory is a recurring theme because it is relevant to every facet of memory. In instances of memory loss, we'll go into the diagnostic steps necessary to find the root cause of the memory problem. More often than not, a helpful treatment is available that is capable of reversing the memory loss and many of the symptoms that go with it.

Keep in mind, however, that human memory is highly subjective and fragile. As you age, you may begin to have some difficulty in remembering, for example, names, particularly when your catalogue or library of memories is very extensive. But if your brain is free from disease or injury, your vital memory should remain intact even into advanced old age.

To make certain that you understand the memory process, I want to discuss in a general way the components of memory so that you can tell the difference between the more and less essential aspects of remembering. I'll also try to give you some information that will help you enhance your ability to remember, even if something has already happened to you to decrease your memory.

I've been fortunate to participate in a revolution in medical science which has brought about major breakthroughs in treating people for loss of vital memory. Thirty years ago I witnessed countless numbers of persons who came to the hospitals where I worked in search of cures for their memory complaints, many of which we were then unable to diagnose, let alone treat. Today a majority of persons with memory problems can be helped. We now know, with certainty, that not all memory loss is permanent, and that there are specific treatments and therapies that can have enormously beneficial results in reversing many kinds of memory loss.

4

What Is Vital Memory?

1

How Vital Memory Controls Life

MEMORY IS the most important mental ability we have. It endows us with the facility to learn new things — in fact, it is an essential part of all new learning — and it influences the development of individual behavior. I'm sure you are aware of the fact that some of us have naturally superior language skills, or mathematical ability, or musical and artistic talents. Even athletic skills are dependent on certain kinds of brain development. But without the capacity to remember, none of those innate skills and talents would be of any use.

Superimposed on genetic endowment, which expresses itself in the structure of the brain and its functional and electrochemical powers, is the fact that the brain changes in response to experiences. This ability of the brain to change with experience is called plasticity. And the fact that the brain does change, allowing our behavior to be modified by cues in our surroundings, is a function of memory. The memories laid down by experience influence current and future behavior.

By these environmental cues I mean not only visual and auditory signals — that is, the signals received by the brain through sight and sound — but also the influences of touch, smell, and taste. When these cues are received in the brain, even though they may be largely in one of the five forms of

7

sensation, mixing or integration always occurs, resulting in a composite record of the whole experience. This record is stored chemically in brain tissue. It becomes a physical part of the brain, and is in fact what we call a memory.

The storage site in the brain varies depending on the predominant sensation of the memory. When you remember a beautiful painting you saw in someone's house, that visual memory is related to the visual cortex of the brain. Likewise, a song you heard on the radio, the sound of a young child's laughter, the noise of an airplane taking off are all auditory memories stored in the auditory cortex. The brain also has specific storage sites for other types of memories.

When I say that memory is the central factor that endows us with the ability to learn, I'm talking about the images and impressions of experiences which are sent to the brain by various sense organs, including the senses of vision and hearing, and which give our surroundings life and meaning. The brain's structure is genetically determined, but even on a microscopic level there is evidence that plasticity as a response to environmental stimuli influences the organization of the brain. As a result of this influence, individual behavior, emotional response, and personality develop in a unique way. That's what differentiates one person from another.

Vital memory is the core or center of the memory process, and it is usually the most protected part of memory. Other more superficial types of memory can decrease before vital memory begins to fail. For example, if individuals have had strokes or head injuries, they may have difficulty with vision and even visual memories. But they can nevertheless retain their basic personalities, carry out many functions completely, and lead almost normal lives.

The brain injuries or diseases that alter or destroy some part of vital memory are always severe. Vital memory includes the memories that are laid down earliest in life, such as the knowledge that allows us to live independently and carry out the essential activities of daily living. These memories tell us when it is appropriate to sleep and when to be awake; how and when to get food and drink so that we can sustain our nutritional requirements; where and when to carry out our functions of elimination in a socially acceptable fashion; how to dress ourselves so that we look appropriate in various contexts; how to cross a street without getting hit by a car (quite a complicated undertaking, requiring knowledge of when and where to cross the street as well as some appreciation of the volume and rules of traffic).

Vital memory is necessary in following the rules of safety so that we dispose of smoking materials, avoid fire, and take into account other factors in our surroundings that are likely to be injurious or dangerous. In other words, vital memory is closely tied to basic brain mechanisms necessary for self-preservation. It helps us to know when to fight or run away in the face of danger. And it helps us gauge the appropriateness of our responses in stressful circumstances.

Vital memory contributes to other kinds of behavior. It is important in generating the learned and remembered responses we have to members of our families and the persons we associate with closely every day. It plays an important role in the give-and-take of social conversation and helps us develop the conditioned responses that determine our emotional tone in various situations — for example, our responses to speech or physical contacts from friends or family. Vital memory helps us to adapt and form appropriate social relations, even when we are confronted by strangers.

Finally, vital memory is at the center of all those memories that summarize our life experiences, from our earliest recollections to the present. Taken as a whole, an inventory of these memories lets us know ourselves — who we are and how we fit into our world. Even more important, they define how we became the individuals we are, with our strengths and vulnerabilities, and with our unique personalities and modes of behavior. In other words, the dynamic memories of our past — of who we are — are with us constantly and influence our responses to almost every challenge we face each day, from the time we awaken until we go to sleep. And even then we don't escape them, because they also shape our dreams.

As you go through the following chapters you should compare the kind of memory difficulties you're having with the memory problems that occur when vital memory is impaired. For the most part, I'm sure, you'll conclude that your memory problems are less serious than the ones I discuss. You know the way to the store, for example, and you don't walk carelessly into traffic. It is losses of vital memory such as these which cause elderly people to lose their orientation. Relatives worry that they'll go outside and try to cross in the middle of busy streets or against stoplights and get hurt or killed. These "wanderers" fill many of the places in nursing homes in the United States.

I'd also like you to remember, however, that even when people get to this stage of losing vital memory — when it is decided they are beyond all hope and they're committed to an institution — it may not be the end of the road for them. The sad fact is that many so-called wanderers have brain or bodily disease that affects brain function. But it is sometimes the case that their loss of vital memory, once its cause is discovered, is not only treatable but also completely reversible. Miracle cures are not required; specific therapies are available that can be used successfully to bring people back to live normal lives, therapies that recoup lost vital memory when symptoms are caused by one of the treatable forms of brain injury or disease.

Never just assume that if memory goes, it is gone forever. Literally scores of different conditions can result in a person's losing all or part of vital memory, conditions that are treatable and reversible. The important point to remember is that the problem or condition causing memory loss has to be identified. A rational course of treatment or prevention cannot begin until the problem has been precisely identified. If the problem is treatable, much can be done. And keep in mind, new information and better treatments are being developed every year.

If you're wondering if you or someone else has a reversible memory loss problem, one that is susceptible to some of the newer treatments, there are a number of ways to improve your chances of a successful outcome. The first step is for an accurate and complete history to be taken in order to provide a clear explanation of the symptoms. When did the memory loss begin? Is the memory loss selective — that is, can the person no longer remember the name of an old friend but still recognize people whom he or she comes in contact with every day? Or is it just the opposite: do ancient memories remain while the person has trouble with recent memory? Memory is like a complex machine with many intricate components. If there's a malfunction, it helps greatly to know just which part isn't working.

To that end, it's important that you understand more about memory so that if and when you do talk with someone about fixing a problem, you'll be able to comprehend better what the problem is. This book will help you understand memory loss and guide you to find the kind of help you need for your specific difficulty. In the next chapters we take a brief look at the memory process and how to test for a memory problem before we discuss ways of diagnosing and reversing memory loss.

2

The Memory Process

ONE OF THE REASONS it's so difficult to understand memory — its mechanisms and what influences it most — is the fact that it is a brain function that is hidden from view. It can't be studied and analyzed, for example, the way we might study how our hands move. Furthermore, the experts who study memory, behavioral neurologists and neuropsychologists, use slightly different terms to describe the same mechanisms, so the vocabulary is confusing.

Behavioral neurologists, for instance, often talk about the memory process, by which they mean ways of holding information that exceeds an individual's attention span. Memories are physically encoded in the chemistry of brain tissue, forming what are known as *engrams*. According to behavioral neurologists, encoding means converting environmental cues into physical, anatomical changes. They talk about "chunking" — how the brain divides complex information so that it can be more easily assimilated and understood — and "linking" — relating environment, all the cues that surround the information that is memorized, to emotions.

Neuropsychologists, by contrast, describe the memory process somewhat differently. They claim that a memory trace is laid down in the brain, and whether it is a shallow trace that is easily forgotten or a deep trace that the mind holds long afterward is related to the emotional content or other related environmental stimuli and the intensity of those stimuli.

I look at the memory process in still another way. I agree with the notion of a holistic environmental record, an integrated mixture of data from our senses of vision, hearing, taste, smell, and touch to form an image, a word, a number, or even an idea or concept. But whether our brains take in these records or not depends on our concentration — our focus of attention. If you are distracted, it is less likely that such a record will enter your brain. If it does, but your concentration is not intense, the event will produce either a shallow memory trace or a weak engram not stored very securely and probably soon forgotten.

It has been argued by some that every event in our lives is indelibly etched in our brains at one level or another. To support this claim some investigators have shown that under hypnosis a subject can remember details of a crime, for example, that he or she was not aware of — say, the license plate number or appearance of the getaway car. But the fact is that memory is selective, and not every detail is remembered.

I do agree that certain things can rivet the attention and make it more likely that a strong memory will be retained. If an event is emotionally charged — that is, if it is associated with anger or fear — or if it is connected with a strong stimulus such as a very pleasant or unpleasant odor or taste, or a loud noise, or a striking visual image, it is more likely to be retained for a long period of time in our memory banks.

There is a good reason why such stimuli are remembered. The limbic or emotional portion of the brain, particularly the part of the limbic brain where the perception of smell is centered, is closely related to the memory circuits in the temporal lobes, the fore part of the brain on either side to the

13

level of the ears. When this part of the brain is activated, the electrochemical mechanisms associated with memory are likely to be more intense, and the memory traces tend to be more enduring.

Memory Aids

For your information, just so you'll be aware of what they are and how they work, I'll briefly explain some memory aids. Many books are available which teach you how to have a better memory for lists of items or people's names, and the following description is not meant to be all-inclusive or complete.

Books that teach you how to have a better memory often take advantage of linking as a factor in the memory process. In fact, the field of mnemonics, linking or associating new data to be remembered with images or other known information, is well recognized by psychologists.

Associating objects to be remembered with images is one of the easiest forms of memory building. Here's how it works. If, for example, you're going to the grocery store and want to buy peanut butter, jelly, lettuce, salad dressing, onions, bread, and syrup, you can remember the items on your list by linking them with "pegs" that you've previously memorized, which represent numbers from one to ten. If your first peg is, for example, a shoe and the first item on your list is peanut butter, you might imagine peanut butter spread all over a shoe. In a similar fashion you would then form separate and unusual images for each item you need to remember. Another method of linking is called acronym building. As you know, an acronym is a word that is formed from the first letters of words, such as ASAP for "as soon as possible," or ZIP code for "zone improvement plan" code. Pegs and acronyms are the easiest memory aids to learn to use, and the simplest. If you have trouble remembering people's names or

14

items on shopping lists, I encourage you to read one of the many excellent books on memory improvement at your bookstore or library.

Concentration, Hypnosis, and Sleep

The key to making any memory system work is concentration, which opens the mind to environmental cues and other information. It is a seeming paradox that persons in a state of hypnosis can get and learn new information and keep it after they have come out of the hypnotic state. This phenomenon is called posthypnotic suggestion. Hypnosis is itself a form of hyperconcentration in which extraneous stimuli have been excluded; it is very different from sleep, and claims that certain methods allow learning while sleeping are unfounded. Once an individual has gone through the rapid eye movement stage into the deeper stages of sleep, the chance of meaningful stimuli reaching the memory circuits and being remembered is slight because concentration and attention-focusing mechanisms are very diminished.

To sum up, I don't believe people in deep stages of sleep can remember information from their surroundings. They are simply unable to focus their attention or concentrate enough to enable most environmental cues to enter the brain in any meaningful way.

Memory Storage

Once memories are encoded, they are stored in the brain. The storage process, according to behavioral neurologists, has two mechanisms: consolidation, that is, the transferring of new information into permanent storage in the brain; and organization and reassemblage of memories when they're called on by ongoing activity or the will of the individual.

I call this whole mechanism of storage the memory bank.

15

Although it is often spoken of as having its locus in a single spot in the brain, the memory bank is actually distributed among a number of parts. Visual memories, for example, are located near the visual centers of the brain, auditory memories near the hearing centers of the brain, and so on. Thus, specific brain injuries or strokes in the visual centers can impair visual memories without causing much reduction of vital memory. Brain injuries or diseases of the memory bank system which do impair or obliterate vital memory must be very extensive in both hemispheres of the brain or very deep within the brain, or both. Fortunately, such damage is uncommon.

Memory Retrieval

The last stage of the memory process is memory retrieval, which involves not only scanning for memories but also their reassemblage or reconstitution in our minds. There are two distinct aspects of memory retrieval. The first is an almost instantaneous process that occurs when challenges to our safety arise. If someone throws something at us, for example, we will immediately duck out of the way — a behavior we may not have practiced in many years, since the days we took part in snowball fights, but the memory is still there. The point is, we don't just stand there and allow ourselves to be hit.

The second, more complicated mechanism involves the willed retrieval of memories. As our memory banks become filled with a catalogue of various memories, those engrams we haven't used in a long time may be difficult to retrieve. I'm sure you've had the same experience I've had of trying to recall the name of someone I haven't seen in years, or even perhaps only a few months. It can elude me so completely that I finally give up and stop thinking about it. Then, a few minutes to a few hours later, the name will pop into my head. The retrieval mechanism was still working; it just took a while to be effective.

One of the reasons it is important for someone giving a speech to practice it before the actual delivery, even when it's meant to be rather extemporaneous, is that the act of practicing allows the person to refurbish the memories that surround the subject of the speech. It puts the memory bank on notice that those memories should be close to the surface for retrieval.

Ronald Reagan presents a good example of how retrieval works — and doesn't work. While he was president, Reagan would diligently review the subjects he would cover in his press conferences, mentally practicing short statements on the various topics. He did exceptionally well for a man in his mid-seventies. Yet in a deposition given in 1990 he was asked questions he had not prepared for, and he then found himself in the embarrassing predicament of not being able to remember even the name of, for example, the chairman of the Joint Chiefs of Staff. To us mere mortals such a lapse seems amazing — after all, the chairman of the Joint Chiefs is a very prestigious figure. But look at it from Reagan's point of view. As president he dealt with hundreds of powerful and prestigious people every day. Once he stopped being president and returned to private life, he had other projects he was involved in, mostly matters not associated with his presidency. Without continual practice and review, it's not surprising his retrieval process wasn't efficient.

The moral to this story is, don't become impatient with yourself when the retrieval process takes longer than you'd like. If you have a large memory bank with a substantial catalogue of memories, don't expect all of them to pop to the surface without some effort on your part to concentrate and make the memories you need available.

Different Kinds of Memory: Art, Music, Athletic Ability

Up to this point in our discussion of the mechanisms of memory we've been focusing on memories related to language and words. But of course there are a number of different kinds of memory, just as there are different kinds of intelligence. People who play musical instruments are well aware of their ability to memorize pieces of music, retaining memories that have little to do with words and in fact are probably in a different hemisphere of the brain.

In one of its forms, Alzheimer's disease severely affects verbal abilities and verbal memories. I remember seeing a fifty-two-year-old insurance salesman from Denver whose career was interrupted by rapidly progressing Alzheimer's. Much of his vital memory was lost, and he almost had to be led around by his wife. A CAT scan showed that he had a very large loss of tissue, particularly in the speech centers in the left, or dominant, hemisphere of his brain. But just looking at the man's x rays and assessing his speech abilities gave a misleading evaluation of his overall potential. When he was seated at the piano, for example, he could still give a creditable rendition of some difficult pieces of both classical and popular music. His musical ability was obviously not impaired.

Similarly, artistic abilities and memories can be preserved even though verbal memory is quite deficient. I would like to see a controlled experiment done in nursing homes in the United States, many of which have large populations of Alzheimer's victims with severe loss of verbal memory. The walls of the rooms of Alzheimer's patients would be adorned with colorful paintings or perhaps simply soothing colors, while speakers piped in relaxing or stimulating music, depending on what response was desired. The study would compare patients given visual and auditory (artistic and musical) stimulation with similar patients who were not to see if the former patients required as much medication, if they were as uncomfortable, and if their general level of function deteriorated as quickly, including their ability to attend to their basic physical needs. My guess is that the nursing home patients who had a more stimulating environment would require less medication.

Muscular and even athletic abilities have a memory component to them. If an athlete in a competitive sport, particularly one facing an adversary, has a deterioration in memory of the responses required to counteract his or her opponent, performance deteriorates. Produced by conditioned responses, habits only become habitual because of the memory process. When muscular coordination or motor habits are interfered with because of a loss of memory, performance will deteriorate.

I myself think that the motor or performance habits are extremely susceptible to memory loss, and that such deterioration occurs in participants in athletic contests even when their strength and reflex speed seem to be unimpaired. Athletic memories have such immediacy that only a slight deterioration may result in a large decrease in performance.

How Doctors Examine the Memory Process

The brain is not a *tabula rasa,* or clean slate, written on by experience. It is a mechanism with inherent capacities for locomotion; autonomic regulation of breathing, heart rate, and blood pressure; and certain feeding abilities, along with genetically acquired traits that manifest themselves as the central nervous system develops. These inherent abilities of the nervous system are molded and shaped by the environment, however, and the molding and shaping — which is a type of learning — are an important aspect of memory. Once memories are formed, they are incorporated into brain structure by physicochemical alterations.

It is impossible to dissociate the brain from its surroundings after environmental stimuli have been laid down as memories in various parts of the brain tissue. This process involves the electrical transmissions from one nerve cell to another in the brain and the chemical changes that take place within and around brain cells. These changes are mediated by special kinds of chemicals called neurotransmitters.

Doctors have learned about the relationship of memory to specific portions of the brain by examining the brains of patients who have died from diseases that produce memory loss. Post-mortem examinations of persons with Korsakoff's psychosis, for example, which is associated with alcoholism and vitamin B-1 deficiency, have shown that the loss of recent memory caused by the disease is related to a lesion in the thalamus. We also know from examining the brains of people who have had loss of recent memory caused by brain injury, or in some cases by symmetrical brain strokes or cerebral infarctions, that lesions of the temporal lobes, especially in the inner anterior portion, may produce such memory loss if the lesions occur on both sides of the brain. One famous case confirmed this discovery. When a neurosurgeon took out both inner anterior portions of the temporal lobes to treat epilepsy, he cured the epilepsy but produced a dramatic loss of recent memory which did not improve.

New Medical Instruments and Their Uses

New instruments have recently been developed which help doctors measure various abnormalities of the brain and correlate them with brain activity and memory. One such instrument is a computerized brain wave machine that records and maps brain waves on a replica of the head. CAT (computerized axial tomography) scans of the brain — a type of x ray which lets us examine the brain tissue as well as the surrounding bone — allow us to see the anatomical structure of the brain and its abnormalities. Using this technique we have been able to learn much more about how brain structures work, and we are now able to correlate destructive changes with losses of recent memory.

Yet another tool available to brain researchers is magnetic resonance imaging (MRI), which, like the CAT scan, allows us to visualize the anatomical structure of the brain. Magnetic resonance imaging works by passing a powerful electromagnetic field over the head, disturbing that field with a radio-frequency beam, and then recording the changes that follow.

Still more recently we've been able to look at the function of brain tissue three-dimensionally by taking tomographic sections through the brain after a patient has been injected with radioactive isotopes. In this technique, known as positron emission tomography, or PET, scanning, abnormal or unusual concentrations of radioactive isotopes can be detected to give a picture of changes in brain function. PET scans produce a color-intensity picture showing areas of increased metabolism in red and less active portions in blue or purple.

Not only are PET scans used to detect abnormalities in people with brain problems, but they also give us fascinating insights into some aspects of brain function in normal volunteer subjects. When an individual tested by such a technique is told, for example, to concentrate visually, that is, to look at a particular object, the visual cortex in the back of the brain lights up. When the subject is asked to listen to a particular sound, the auditory centers in the inner part of the temporal lobes light up. When the individual is given a task requiring substantial thinking, portions of the frontal lobes light up. And when a subject is asked to remember a visual object, metabolism increases not only in the visual cortex but also in portions of the temporal lobes, those parts we've already indicated are important in memory function. Such scans make a rather striking picture of at least some memory functions, giving us hope that we may be able to trace certain kinds of brain function more accurately in the future with similar techniques.

3

Memory Testing

WHAT KINDS of memory loss are serious enough for you to consult a neurologist about? What memory symptoms should you look for in yourself or your relatives which are of real concern? The short answer is that any memory problem that is persistent or severe enough to cause you to worry about it should send you to your doctor. Even if it proves to be inconsequential, it's worth your while to know that it isn't serious, and finding that out should shield you from needless anxiety and the secondary depression that can make a trivial memory problem into a disabling symptom.

But aren't some memory symptoms more important than others, symptoms that demand more medical attention and formal memory testing? Yes, but they vary in degree and seriousness. For example, if someone is able to drive the same route every day for years without difficulty and suddenly begins to get lost, that's a sign that formal memory testing and neurological or neuropsychological testing should be done. If someone you know tells the same story over and over again, and does so even after telling the story less than an hour before, memory testing is mandatory. If someone has a pattern of forgetfulness which is progressive and disabling to the point that memory loss interferes with job performance or basic functioning, memory testing is imperative.

Mind you, the situations I've described do not involve forgetting things like items on a shopping list, where you put your keys, or someone's name. But as I've said, any memory symptoms that cause you anxiety should be looked into, to prevent unnecessary worry and worsening of the symptoms. Whether it is done by a neurologist or a neuropsychologist, memory testing is the most important initial diagnostic step to separate serious complaints from trivial ones.

Before I describe specific memory tests, it is useful to point out that the memory abilities each of us is born with, or ultimately develops, differ. Some of us have better musical memory, or artistic memory, or athletic memory. Some of us have a very fine mathematical or scientific memory, whereas others are especially endowed with good verbal memory. Regardless of what the ability is, as a rule the more a memory function is used, the better preserved it will be as we grow older — as long as the memory function in the brain is not weakened by brain injury or brain disease.

As we grow older, we generally experience what is known as benign memory loss, which means, for one thing, that many of us have difficulty remembering individuals' names. Several studies have indicated that older people have difficulty in short-term learning and with short-term memory, but these problems don't occur in everyone. Studies reviewed by Robert Katzman and Robert D. Terry, for example, showed that fourteen people who had taken a test of mental efficiency and were then retested thirty-five years later, when they were between sixty and seventy-four years old, had unchanged or even slightly improved vocabulary scores. Their overall learning scores, however, decreased from an average of seventeen to an average of thirteen (on a scale of zero to twenty), and the results of retention tests declined from eighteen to thirteen over the thirty-five-year period. But there were wide differences among subjects, and those who were not hypertensive exhibited no decline in their memory scores over a ten-year period.

One reason older people may not do as well as younger ones on memory tests is that they may not have been taught to use various mnemonic techniques in new learning. What one is really measuring, then, is a cultural rather than a physiological phenomenon of the brain.

Of course, memory is an important part of all new learning. In order to find out whether a person's memory is functioning at optimal level it is necessary to perform tests, both simple and elaborate, of learning and memory abilities. Typically, either a psychologist or a neuropsychologist is the trained medical professional who does such testing. I won't include an entire test here since it would be far too long and detailed for you to use. But I will explain what is usually tested for, and why, so that you'll understand the importance of these tests in determining the cause of reversible memory loss.

Auditory and Visual Testing

One of the most common ways in which a neuropsychologist tests memory is to see how rapidly a given subject can learn visual or auditory information. Data are presented, for example, in the form of cards showing words or pictures. The subject is given a limited period of time to study these cards and is then asked to recall the information after one, two, or three repetitions.

Auditory learning is tested in the same way, with verbal instructions presented regarding words, phrases, or ideas. After suitable delays, and at times with repetitions and cues, the subject is asked to repeat the information in either writing or speech. These tests evaluate not only a person's visual and auditory memory but also other aspects of intelligence and language function.

25

A Neurological Memory Test

As a neurologist, I usually divide memory testing into three parts to correspond with the three major aspects of memory: immediate recall, recent memory, and ancient (or remote) memory.

When I test immediate recall I'm not only testing immediate memory but also an individual's attention span. For example, I will give someone seven numbers — 5, 6, 8, 4, 3, 2, 7 — and ask the person to repeat them. Then I will give the same individual five numbers and have the person repeat those in reverse order. Keep in mind that people with severe deficiencies in recent-memory ability can still repeat numbers or phrases like "no ifs, ands, or buts" if their attention spans are of normal duration.

Testing of recent memory gives a more penetrating assessment of memory abilities. Here I ask the subject to remember the names of three or four unrelated objects, such as a table, a flower, and a book, but I don't allow the person being tested to keep repeating the list over and over in his or her mind. If I did that I wouldn't be testing recent memory; I'd be back at immediate memory or immediate recall. What I do is intersperse my questions about the list items with a number of other questions which focus attention on another topic. For example, I give various instructions, I ask mathematical questions, I ask the subject to interpret proverbs, I ask geographical questions, and I make the questions difficult enough so that the person's mind cannot revert to the original words that are supposed to be remembered. Then, after three and a half to four minutes, I ask the subject to repeat the three or four words in the same sequence I gave them. The point of this test of recent memory is that it demands that a person be able to hold information exceeding his or her attention span for the words to be remembered.

Ancient memory testing is somewhat trickier. At one time I used to test ancient memory by asking patients questions about geography: for example, What states border Massachusetts? Now, however, if I test persons under the age of thirty-five, they probably won't be able to tell me — not because of their deficient memories but rather because of their deficient education, since geography is rarely taught in our public school systems anymore.

Because presidents and often past presidents are figures in the news, and because most people at one time or another watch television news, I usually test ancient, or remote, memory by having the subject give me the name of the current president followed by that of preceding presidents. Again, older patients seem to do better on this test than younger ones, who complain, "Well, of course, I wasn't alive when Truman or Eisenhower was president." What they're really telling me is that American history was not taught effectively in their schools.

Ancient memory is best tested through those memories we all have in common. It is very difficult to get a valid test of remote memory by asking people about the events of their private lives without independent verification from relatives — and even so, the information gathered in this way may be misleading since "normal" family members can have widely differing views on how a specific event or story unfolded. Also, individuals with severe damage to the inner parts of both anterior temporal lobes, who have great difficulty with recent memory and in learning new information, also make up stories. If you ask them about events in their private lives in order to test remote memory, they may give a very complete account that is nevertheless absolutely false.

Such was the case with George, a thirty-eight-year-old social science teacher at a Boston high school, who had a benign tumor in the center of his brain. By benign I mean that it was not cancerous, it did not metastasize, and it didn't invade the surrounding brain, but it produced symptoms because it pressed on sensitive areas of the brain. As the tumor grew

27

larger it could not be treated with deep x-ray therapy alone, and therefore as much of it as possible had to be removed surgically.

George had severe loss of recent memory before the operation, and although the tumor was removed almost in its entirety, it had already caused enough damage to central brain structures that his loss of recent memory persisted in the postoperative period. If I went to see him in his room, for example, he would talk to me quite pleasantly. But if I were called away for a minute or two and then came back into the room, he would not remember that he had just seen me. He would greet me all over again as though it were a completely new conversation, and he would swear that he had never seen me before. He was absolutely convinced that he was telling the truth.

In addition, George told me about his life experiences in the most exaggerated terms. Rather than a high school teacher, he implied he was a famous college professor and lecturer (perhaps his secret ambition); he also said he was married and had four lovely children. Our investigations failed to disclose that he had ever been married or had any children.

Even though he described his past life in great detail, my conversation with his elderly parents failed to substantiate any of his claims. He was, in fact, demonstrating the symptoms of confabulation. This false reporting of remote memory occurs in many diseases that involve the center of the brain, in an area called the thalamus and hypothalamus. Not only tumors but also hemorrhages, strokes, and nutritional deficiencies such as an insufficient amount of thiamine, or vitamin B-1, in the diet (a deficiency associated with alcohol abuse) often produce this syndrome. George wasn't purposefully trying to deceive me or anyone else. But because of his condition, he remembered his life as having been very different from what it was, and far more successful. With the removal of the tumor and subsequent deep x-ray treatments, however, he gradually regained some of his memory abilities, although his recollection of much of his childhood and school years did not return.

To sum up, since neurologists and neuropsychologists can't rely on personal memories in testing remote-memory ability, they will carry out tests for information that should have been learned in school or that is part of our historical or political heritage.

Let me assure you first that if your immediate recall, recent memory, and remote memory are normal, it is unlikely that you have anything to worry about as far as vital memory functions are concerned. Also, if you do have some problems in memory testing, it doesn't necessarily mean you are suffering from an incurable brain disease. In fact, it may mean that you simply need to have a good medical and neurological assessment. There are many treatable causes of memory loss, and such loss can be promptly reversed with effective therapy, which I will describe in later chapters.

As we look at examples of memory problems in various persons, you will see that the pattern of memory loss in each is significant and that these different patterns can be discovered and diagnosed by various mental status and psychological tests. Individuals who are agitated or depressed may have a variable pattern in their memory tests, as was the case with Gary, forty-three, a restaurant manager who came to see me after he began to forget lists of items he was going to the supermarket to buy.

Gary's memory was so bad, he told me, that he even forgot to kiss his wife when he left for work. His memory tests did show areas of memory lapse, both visual and auditory. Some mistakes in recent memory were made, and some in remote recall. But Gary also had islands of memory proficiency which were outstanding. He would remember the list of objects in the test of recent memory very well on one occasion and not at all on another. He could remember the names of only three presidents on one test occasion, but rattled off the names of seven mayors of Boston in reverse order with ease.

This variable test pattern indicated a disorder like mild depression, not stroke or Alzheimer's, as the cause of Gary's problem, and this problem was eminently treatable. By contrast, Hank, a fifty-one-year-old department store salesman, wasn't himself at all concerned about memory loss; it was his relatives who insisted he come to see me. They complained that he kept telling the same old stories to them over and over, sometimes after only fifteen-minute intervals. Hank also got so lost when he was driving that they no longer allowed him to be in a car alone.

Memory testing showed that Hank's results were consistent; repeated tests of recent memory showed him to be very deficient. He also had greater difficulty with material presented visually than with verbal information. The test results didn't necessarily mean that Hank's memory deficiencies were untreatable, but they did show that he had a serious problem requiring complete neurological and medical evaluations. In the next chapter we'll look at what these evaluations consist of, and how someone like Hank can be helped.

Reversal of Memory Loss

4

Reversible Causes of Memory Loss and Their Treatment

Where Does It Begin?

HAVE YOU NOTICED that as you've gotten older you've become more set in your ways? Well, it's hardly surprising then that your father and mother, or grandparents if they're still alive, have the same problem. If they had poor memories when they were young, their memories may have become terrible in their advanced years. But is this problem just a function of getting older, or is it a medical condition for which they should be receiving treatment? Do their memory problems indicate a brain abnormality? And, more important, are their problems treatable and reversible?

When my grandfather had severe memory loss in his eighties resulting from Alzheimer's disease, I was tempted to look back at the symptoms of personality change that had occurred ten to fifteen years before the disease was diagnosed. Did those symptoms indicate the beginning of Alzheimer's? The more I thought about it the more I was sure that they probably did not. The changes he went through were more likely related to his grief over the death of his wife of more than forty years than anything else.

Memory loss in an elderly person may begin in such a subtle or gradual fashion that the resulting personality change or disability is difficult to differentiate from the more usual day-to-day fluctuations in performance. It can manifest itself in such things as missing meals, with weight loss or malnutrition, or a change in dressing habits, neatness, cleanliness, or hygiene. Are these reasons to seek medical help, considering that the elderly person is likely to react angrily to the suggestion that he or she should see a doctor about any of these problems?

In younger people, memory loss may appear suddenly, especially after a head injury or a bout of alcohol or drug abuse. Sometimes it occurs after someone is put on medication for sleeplessness or anxiety, which results from depression. Should anyone with these problems seek medical attention?

The decision about whether someone has a genuine memory deficiency is not an easy one to make. Even doctors have memory problems, so don't be discouraged if this gray area between brain abnormalities and social or psychological influences seems confusing and imprecise. It is. There are, however, some things we can do to help.

First, we can sort out the memory complaints that do not usually indicate serious brain difficulties and are unlikely to require examination by a physician. It is, of course, not uncommon or unusual for anyone to have trouble remembering things from time to time. If you have any of the following problems, in the absence of any other symptoms, you most likely do not need to consult a doctor:

• forgetting names
• misplacing keys, glasses, or other small items
• not being able to find your car in a parking lot
• not being able to remember items to shop for at the store
• not being able to recognize someone in an unfamiliar setting

What follows is a list of memory problems and the changes that occur in function and personality. These symptoms do require medical investigation:

- getting lost while driving a familiar route
- completely forgetting important appointments
- telling the same stories over and over to the same people during a short space of time (i.e., no short-term recall)
- having periods of confusion over what time it is or where one is
- being unable to manage a checkbook or take care of simple finances
- experiencing a sudden or gradual change in personality
- having difficulty with language (e.g., naming objects)
- experiencing a sudden change in artistic or musical ability
- undergoing a loss of memory which is disabling to the point that work is impossible or one's daily activity level is upset

To answer questions about the significance of memory loss, whether in the young or the old, more fully, you or a friend or relative can carry out some preliminary testing for yourself (or on each other). The following self-help test of mental status will help you determine if an examination by a neurologist is necessary. The steps are simple on paper, but they may be difficult to carry out if the person you suspect may have a memory problem is much older than you are; if you are both unsure of your motives and become defensive or uncooperative; or if either of you is too confused to follow the instructions or is humiliated by the testing process.

If you can't complete all of the test, respond to as many of the entries as you can. Sometimes subjects' responses, even when they aren't right, can give others an intuitive feeling about the significance of their memory difficulties.

Here is the sample test:

1. Give your friend or relative three words to remember — for example, table, lamp, flower — and ask that they be repeated after five minutes of doing other mental tasks.
2. See whether your friend knows what the date is and where exactly you both are.
3. Have the person repeat the phrase "No ifs, ands, or buts."
4. Have the person name and identify common objects — for example, a ring, a pencil, glasses, and the like.
5. Ask the person to draw the face of a clock and put the numbers in the proper positions.
6. Have the person subtract sixteen from one hundred and multiply thirteen by twelve.
7. Ask the person to interpret the proverb "A stitch in time saves nine."
8. Have your friend name the current president of the United States and the preceding six presidents in reverse order.
9. Have him or her read a paragraph from a book, magazine, or newspaper and explain what the passage means.
10. Ask the person to name the states that border your state.

You might wonder why this kind of formal testing is necessary if you already suspect that the person you're worried about has a problem. Since you've observed your friend's muddled thinking and memory problems at close range, isn't that enough? The answer is that your subjective impressions, or even the impressions of a trained professional, such as a doctor, may turn out to be wrong. Testing done in the manner described above — that is, formal testing of mental status — gives some objective basis for a decision about what's wrong.

If your friend or relative "passes" this simple test, the person probably doesn't need to see a neurologist, despite complaints about poor memory. But if your friend cannot respond accurately to all the questions, it may be that his or her degree of memory loss and personality change is significant. It is important to carry out neurological testing in anyone who has suffered genuine memory loss and personality change, whatever the person's age — but more especially in those who are elderly. My own clinical investigations of elderly people with personality change and beginning memory loss, however, often reveal no evidence of Alzheimer's disease but rather clinical problems that are the result of some other cause — one that is frequently treatable.

Danny, seventy-nine, was referred by one of my physician acquaintances to the center I co-founded for the treatment of memory impairment. His daughter was very worried about his living alone because when she visited him he often seemed bewildered. Danny would, for example, open the cellar door of his house rather than the closet door to put his coat away. He also became confused whenever he drove to the next state to visit his daughter.

He was a retired real estate broker and scoutmaster who had no demands on his time. And because he lived alone he was careless about preparing meals and sometimes didn't eat much for two or three days at a time.

From his medical history, I had anticipated that he might be a candidate for enrollment in a therapeutic trial of an anti-Alzheimer's drug. But even minimal testing showed that his mental status was much too good for him to be classified as being in the beginning stages of Alzheimer's. In fact, Danny was suffering from depression.

The steps we at the center took with him are the same that would be taken with any elderly person who is failing to thrive, especially one recently widowed or bereaved. First, we got him a dog. Having to care for an animal imposed a routine on Danny's life because the dog had to be fed and walked regularly, and he was a constant companion. Next we insisted that Danny take up being a scoutmaster again. He also reestablished social ties through his church, where he went to at least two functions a week which offered not only nourishing food but companionship. And we got him to start a mild exercise routine, with activities he could easily do on a daily basis. Finally, we contacted his physician, who reviewed the dosages of his medications — particularly the drugs he was taking for hypertension — and gave him a daily menu to help maintain his nutrition.

Danny's prescription to regain mental health should be used by anyone who is beginning to drop out or lose motivation. This is especially true if the person performs well on a mental status test but continues to have memory and other mental symptoms. To generalize the advice I gave to Danny, I recommend the following to anyone in his position:

- Establish a routine. Having a pet, such as a dog, is a good way to do this.
- Reestablish social ties through a church or voluntary organization.
- Make sure meals are nutritious; join Meals on Wheels or some other program if food preparation is a problem.
- Consult your doctor about medications and diet.
- Start a mild exercise program (e.g., brisk walking) if possible.

The above suggestions in no way substitute for medical, psychiatric, or neurological management when it is needed. However, they are an important supplement to any program to maintain well-being for persons with memory symptoms but no neurological or medical disease.

I tell my patients never to give up hope, even if they are given a diagnosis of Alzheimer's disease, because some treatable conditions, like the pseudodementia of depression, can mimic Alzheimer's closely. In the early stages at least, it is almost impossible to tell them apart. If you have any doubt about what is wrong, get a second opinion from a neurologist and follow the clinical steps listed at the end of this chapter.

Competence

No sight is more pathetic than watching relatives squabble over the estate of a victim of memory loss in probate court, attempting to declare him or her incompetent. Psychiatrists hired by one side will say one thing, and psychiatrists on the other side precisely the opposite. The plain truth of the matter is that a diagnosis of Alzheimer's is not equivalent to mental incompetence. And Alzheimer's victims can continue, with assistance, to manage many of their affairs until they have lost significant portions of their vital memories. Finding out whether someone is or isn't competent is by no means a clear-cut process.

What would you do if you or a family member suffered memory loss? In order to determine what the appropriate course of action should be, a number of specific questions need to be asked and answered. For example, do you or anyone in your family have a loss of vital memory? That is, does the person not just forget someone's name or the items on a shopping list, but rather has he or she undergone a loss of orientation? Is the person aware of what happened yesterday? What he or she has to do today? What the prospects for tomorrow are?

If someone in your family has this kind of problem, he or she needs immediate help. But don't assume that the clinical situation is hopeless or that the chances for recovery are slight, because they're not. Several different disorders can cause vital-memory problems, and many of them are easily treatable: such entities as clinical depression, brain poisoning with alcohol or street drugs (including amphetamines, cocaine, barbiturates, marijuana, Angel Dust, and a variety of drugs prescribed by physicians), nutritional problems like malnutrition and dehydration, and a variety of medical and

39

even neurological disorders. Most of these medical conditions can produce some loss of vital memory, but the loss varies depending on the severity of the problem.

Before I discuss some of these problems in detail, let me also point out that there can sometimes be two or more causes for lapses in vital memory, all of which contribute to a loss of intellectual function. For example, a person who has poisoned his or her brain with alcohol may also suffer from a vitamin B-1 deficiency, have had a head injury, and be subject to epileptic seizures. Each of these problems can impair or reduce vital memory.

Sadly, too, many doctors are trained to look only for the chief cause of a problem, and they fail to dig deeper to discover contributing factors. Your best defense against an incomplete diagnosis is to insist on thorough medical testing and analysis. The following paragraphs explain what you need to know and what you should expect from a competent diagnostician.

Doctors Who Investigate Memory Lapses

Doctors come with a variety of labels, but these labels don't tell you much about a physician's competence or diligence. A family physician, or generalist, may be more effective and persistent in diagnostic efforts than a high-powered specialist who looks too narrowly at one symptom and misses an underlying cause or a treatable problem. Many family physicians have special training in internal medicine and geriatrics, and some, like the family physicians at the University of Oklahoma Medical School branch in Tulsa, take a special interest in the diagnosis and treatment of reversible causes of memory loss and dementia.

Geriatricians usually have a background in internal medicine and have been examined in all areas of internal medicine, particularly those dealing with heart and lung disease, liver disease, kidney disease, and rheumatology. Some are very interested in the nervous system and good at the differential diagnosis and treatment of memory loss and dementing illness. Others prefer to focus on diseases of the heart, lungs, or joints. These doctors should refer patients suspected of having dementing illness to a specialist in that area.

Most physicians trained in neurology are well equipped to investigate the causes of memory loss and dementing illness and to carry out appropriate treatment. But some board-certified neurologists are criticized because their clinical interests are so narrow that they may miss a potentially treatable cause of dementing illness. Some neurologists, for example, specialize in muscle diseases and their treatment, and they're not interested in the degenerative diseases of the brain. If a physician doesn't try to find every possible cause of memory loss in making a neurological evaluation, he or she is not the doctor for you. You will need another neurologist.

Psychiatrists come in all shapes and sizes. In recent years the new field of geriatric psychiatry has emerged. Psychiatrists in this field are especially expert in treating depression in the elderly and also in psychopharmacology, the art and science of balancing medications to give the most beneficial effects and the fewest side effects. Most geriatric psychiatrists demand a complete evaluation of a patient's medical and neurological state before they will undertake any definitive treatment. But this is not true of all psychiatrists. Some psychiatrists ignore potentially treatable medical problems and correctable neurological ailments, much to the detriment of their patients' well-being.

Psychologists often treat patients with group psychotherapy or various environmental psychotherapies in the nursing home setting. They also carry out various kinds of psychological testing. They are not physicians, however, and they should not begin a treatment program on any patient with dementing illness until the patient has had a complete medical and neurological evaluation.

41

An Optimal Test of Vital Memory

With these factors in mind, my partner, Tom Sabin, a neurologist, and I began the Center for Memory Impairment and Neurobehavioral Disturbances (CMIND). The center's chief effort was to examine patients with memory loss and disabling dementia, or other forms of behavioral disturbance, before rather than after they were committed to nursing homes. We have also examined many residents of nursing homes to try to find treatable problems, lessen their symptoms, and make the lives of these patients both more comfortable and more rewarding.

One thing we require for every patient is as complete a medical history as possible, and this is often difficult to get. The histories of patients in nursing homes have often been lost, and significant factors may not come to light during a diagnostic evaluation. Second, we do a number of blood tests to screen for various conditions — anemia, malnutrition, diabetes, thyroid impairment, syphilis, electrolyte imbalance — and get appropriate medical evaluations when these tests disclose some problem.

Next we have the patient psychologically tested for evidence of emotional problems such as severe depression. Finally, we take the blood levels of all medications the patient is on which can cause memory loss or other dementing illness. If the patient exhibits some evidence of depression, we have him or her seen by a geriatric psychiatrist for evaluation for psychotherapy or other appropriate therapy.

A neurological examination and if necessary a brain wave test (that is, an electroencephalogram) are done on the patient, along with a visualization of the brain itself in a CAT or MRI scan as well as neuropsychological testing, giving a detailed analysis of memory function. Most important, we have a senior member of our staff correlate the findings from all the examinations. In writing an integrated summary report to the referring physician, this doctor lists the pertinent findings from each examination and offers medical recommendations, which may include a drug "holiday," new medications, psychotherapy, a change in the patient's residence or in his or her relationships with, for example, family members. At times a surgical or operative lesion such as hydrocephalus, a brain tumor, or a blood clot (subdural hematoma) is found pressing on the brain and it must then be removed.

I have not discussed all the tests that might need to be done on each patient. For example, some patients may need a spinal tap or lumbar puncture to look at their spinal fluid. Not every patient needs every test. The evaluation still depends on the physician's knowledge and judgment, but we think the CMIND paradigm is appropriate not only for determining whether a patient should be sent to a nursing home, but for assessing the condition of many patients already in such facilities. I have sent a summary of the tests described here to the doctor in the Health Care Finance Administration (the agency that oversees Medicare in the United States) who is responsible for the regulations concerning the diagnosis and treatment of nursing home patients, in hopes that it will be used in future Medicare guidelines.

National Policy Issues

The present diagnosis and treatment of elderly patients with memory loss is often inadequate, and the medical approach is just part of the answer to a perplexing and difficult problem. Social and economic solutions are also needed, including, for example, intergenerational housing, that is, semidetached housing that would accommodate three generations in a single family. But of course such solutions address a wider problem than memory loss. Nevertheless, memory loss is a salient symptom of the hundreds of thousands of elderly persons who now challenge us to provide better medical and diagnostic treatment centers in the United States.

Needless to say, the more people we can keep out of nursing homes the better. If we can slow down or reverse memory loss, everyone gains. It is important to keep people active and contributing to society, and older individuals, because of the richness of their experience, have much to offer the rest of us. It is doubly necessary that we determine the precise cause of memory loss and dementing illness as quickly as symptoms appear so that appropriate medical steps can be taken. The cost of not doing this, in decreasing the quality of the patient's life as well as increasing the financial burden on all the rest of us, makes any other alternative unthinkable.

Vital Memory Points to Remember

Which memory symptoms are probably not significant?

It is not uncommon or unusual for anyone to have trouble remembering things from time to time. If you have any of the following problems, in the absence of any other symptoms, you most likely do not need to consult a doctor:

- forgetting names
- misplacing keys, glasses, or other small items
- not being able to find your car in a parking lot
- not being able to remember items to shop for at the store
- not being able to recognize someone in an unfamiliar setting

Which memory symptoms do require medical investigation?

If you have any of the following symptoms you should have a medical professional check you out:

- getting lost while driving a familiar route
- completely forgetting important appointments
- telling the same stories over and over to the same people during a short space of time (i.e., no short-term recall)

- having periods of confusion over what time it is or where you are
- being unable to manage a checkbook or take care of simple finances
- experiencing a sudden or gradual change in personality
- having difficulty with language (e.g., naming objects)
- experiencing a sudden change in artistic or musical ability
- undergoing a loss of memory which is disabling to the point that work is impossible or your daily activity level is upset

What should you do if your symptoms require medical investigation?

1. Ask your doctor to refer you to a neurologist. If you don't have a doctor, call your local medical society and ask for a referral to a neurologist specializing in problems of memory loss and dementing illness.
2. When you see the neurologist, make certain that a full mental status examination, *including memory testing,* is done. If the results are not completely normal, the neurologist will refer you to a neuropsychologist for detailed memory testing.
3. If the results of your memory test aren't normal, you will also need a complete physical examination, including blood and urine tests to determine levels of the medications you are on. Furthermore, you will need a complete neurological examination in which a detailed history of your problem, together with an accurate medical history, is taken.
4. If these tests are not completely normal, you should have a CAT or MRI scan of the brain as well as an electroencephalogram and possibly a lumbar puncture. Detailed neuropsychological tests, if not already done, should complete this evaluation.

What should you do if problems arise?

1. If your physician or neurologist is unwilling to have these tests done, you must find a physician who will do them.
2. If the results of these tests are normal and you still have a pattern of memory loss, you should consult a geriatric psychiatrist to establish whether depression is present and, if so, how it should be treated.
3. If your doctor does not sit down with you to review all the medications you are taking and how they might be contributing to your problem, you must find a doctor who will.
4. If after all the above steps are carried out you have symptoms of memory loss and still were not given a diagnosis, you should repeat the evaluation in three to six months.
5. A complete and thorough evaluation should identify the cause of any memory loss. Then, either the loss can be reversed by appropriate treatment or further progression of memory loss can be prevented.
6. Even if a progressive disease like Alzheimer's is found, a number of measures can be taken to prolong the useful life of an Alzheimer's patient, including:
   —diagnosing and treating other causes of dementia which make the symptoms of Alzheimer's worse
   —helping the patient establish and keep a routine around times and places
   —making orienting aids such as large calendars and clocks available
   —allowing the Alzheimer's patient as much freedom as possible compatible with safety (e.g., doors to the outside should be locked, but doors to and from the bathroom or bedroom should stay open)
7. One should always allow Alzheimer's patients to remain as productive as possible for as long as they can function effectively. For example, one Alzheimer's patient con-

stantly got lost coming back from the bathroom but could still make sound decisions about investments. Another patient could hardly talk yet managed to plant a beautiful flower garden. Remember that a person's having a diagnosis of Alzheimer's does not mean that he or she is necessarily incompetent, by either a clinical or a legal definition. The individual's competence depends on the state and extent of brain disease.

5

Depression: The Most Common Cause of Reversible Vital Memory Loss and Intellectual Deterioration

YOU MAY HAVE a poor or failing memory that interferes not only with achievement of your hopes and aspirations but also with your everyday performance. But do you know what is causing your memory difficulty? Although a precise diagnosis often depends on appropriate medical and psychological testing, you can begin to get some idea of the cause by looking at the kind of memory problem you have as well as at some of the other problems in your life which have coincided with your memory loss.

Do you find that you have difficulty learning new things? Do you have difficulty concentrating? Are you easily distracted so that the focus of your attention wavers? In other words, do you have a short attention span? Do you feel that you try to force your mental processes to function efficiently, only to find yourself bogged down like a prize fighter trying to throw a punch under water? Do you feel anxious or have difficulty sleeping? Do you wake up very early in the morning, well before you want to? Do you find yourself worried or upset? Do things look hopeless, as though there is no end to your troubles and you will never be able to work your way out of difficulty? If you are having memory difficulties along with these kinds of symptoms, it is likely that your problem is caused in large part by depression.

An example of this kind of problem was presented by Thelma, a sixty-three-year-old widow, who told me, "Doctor, I can't remember anything. It's a good thing I live right next to the grocery store because I have to go back three or four times a day just to remember the things I was supposed to shop for. I finally started making a list, but then I forgot it and had to go back home to get it."

When I took Thelma's history, it turned out that her problems with memory had started about four weeks before she saw me. This was a tip-off that something that had happened recently changed her level of functioning. More important, no unusual medical problem had arisen to produce this sudden change in her level of competence. So I began to probe her life situation: did she have problems with her children? The answer was no. Thelma assured me that she didn't smoke or drink and had never taken drugs. What about her finances? Well, she lived on a widow's pension and had been just able to get by until about a month before. What happened at that time? She had gotten her property tax bill on her tiny little bungalow; her taxes had gone up dramatically and tipped her precarious money situation toward bankruptcy. She told me, "Doctor, my husband Sam and I worked all our lives to save a little something, and now it's all gone. Now the town is going to take away my house."

My treatment of Thelma was not medical but rather social and political. I got in touch with one of the senior town officials, who told me he would do everything he could to help her. The very fact that something could be done, and was being done, elevated her spirits and improved her level of memory functioning. Thelma had a reversible kind of memory loss, probably the most common and the most easily misdiagnosed one — that is, memory loss associated with depression. There are, in fact, several forms of depression, and all produce some loss of memory and reduction of previous intellectual capacities. But all forms of depression don't act equally to reduce vital memory.

Doctors often classify depression by its severity. No matter what the cause, the most severe forms produce a profound loss of vital memory. The least severe, on the other hand, do not impair vital memory, but other forms of memory may be affected. It shouldn't be surprising that this is the case. Almost all of us know how a feeling of depression can impair our day-to-day functioning. Our efficiency is reduced, we don't pay attention to what people say to us, our personal finances may fall into disarray, paying bills for things like taxes and insurance may not get done, and we stop our routine and may not even get to work.

There are other classifications of depression. Cases related to life adjustment problems are psychological in origin. Doctors frequently observe grief reactions, for example, when patients lose spouses, parents or children, or others who are close to them. Some doctors witness "burnout" syndrome when depressed patients become discouraged with the jobs they're in and don't see any future, or when they are severely stressed by their jobs and find no way of achieving success, looking forward only to increasing demands and unpleasant responsibilities. Such stress-induced depression can often be treated by various forms of psychotherapy or environmental change (for example, changing a job). Often it is self-limited.

Depression in the elderly related to life adjustment problems can be very disabling because many elderly persons lack the resources and the recuperative powers of the young, and moreover their symptoms can mimic dementia and thus be misdiagnosed. In the early stages of the disorder, increased support from relatives and friends may stop the downward slide before the patient goes into deep depression, requiring antidepressants and professional psychotherapy to remedy.

50

Other kinds of depression seem to be related not to a stressful environment but rather to some abnormality in brain chemistry or neurotransmitter function — in other words, to some problem in the brain itself. Sometimes patients who have this kind of depression find that other members of their families — parents, grandparents, brothers, sisters, cousins — have the same complaints. At times the depression is accompanied by severe mood swings; that is, periods of elation and manic activity which are followed by depression. Here too there may be a family history of this disorder, which, strangely enough, is often associated with high intelligence and a record of achievement. Some forms of depression, finally, seem to be related to menopause, which may also trigger neurochemical changes in the brain.

All of these brain-related forms of depression can produce some loss of vital memory, but the important point to remember is that they are treatable, and the lives and memories of patients suffering from these symptoms can be greatly improved. The following sections describe the more typical clinical pictures of depression and vital memory loss, the kind of problem that brings people to hospitals and, if unrecognized and untreated, sends them to nursing homes.

Clinical Depression and Memory Loss

When most of us think of a person who is depressed, we get a mental image of someone who is tearful, slowed down, almost apathetic, not moving much, possibly sitting or lying down, just staring blankly off into space. Although some severely depressed people are like that, many of the ten million persons in the United States who have suffered from clinical depression sometime during their lives behave somewhat differently. They may feel hopeless and have a sense that things are closing in on them. Usually they seem agitated. Sleep disturbances are quite common, and often they wake up early in the morning and can't get back to sleep.

When such persons come to see a doctor they appear to be more anxious than depressed, and it is not uncommon for the doctor to prescribe a tranquilizer and a sleeping pill. Unfortunately, these medications not only don't bring the patient out of the depressed state but may make it much worse.

Billy, a fifty-three-year-old machinist, was one of my patients who had this happen to him. Over a number of years, Billy became more and more concerned about losing his memory. He thought he was following in the steps of his father, who had memory lapses before the age of sixty and who finally suffered profound dementia leading to premature death. Billy had always been an independent sort of person, steady and hard-working, but his life had been beset by troubles. His first wife died of cancer, leaving him with a ten-year-old daughter to raise, and his second marriage was unhappy and finally ended in divorce a month before he came to talk with me.

When I saw him the first thing I noticed was that Billy had trouble relaxing. Everything was in motion — his hands, feet, arms, and torso; he looked like a four-year-old who couldn't sit still. He was playing with his glasses, and he seemed overly sensitive to any change in my mood or manner when I spoke to him. Even though his chief complaint was his memory loss, he also told me that he had trouble sleeping at night and that he woke up at five-thirty in the morning and couldn't get back to sleep. He looked bleary-eyed, and he said his work was deteriorating. On some days he couldn't go to work at all. Finally he admitted that he had been trying to treat his memory problem with increasing amounts of alcohol. (Incidentally, it is extremely common for depressed patients to medicate themselves with alcohol, cocaine, amphetamines, or other street drugs. The initial drug- or alcohol-induced euphoria is often followed by deeper depression, which is even more resistant to subsequent doses of drugs or alcohol.) Of course, the alcohol didn't work; it just made him more depressed as well as alcohol-dependent.

The reason for Billy's depression was fairly obvious from his history. The dissolution of his stormy marriage, his only daughter's living with a semi-alcoholic man, financial troubles, and threatened layoffs at work all contributed to a very real environmental stress–related depression. On top of this, he began to perceive his own mortality as he approached sixty, the age at which his father's mental powers had begun to decline.

Seeing how agitated he was, it would have been the easiest thing in the world to give him some sleeping pills, or Valium, or Ativan. But what he really needed was problem resolution — someone to talk to his boss to find out what his chances for continued employment were (they turned out to be good), and family counseling sessions for him and his daughter. It helped that she was quite sensitive to her father's problems, and even though her living arrangements didn't change to suit him completely, the sessions at least allowed Billy and his daughter to achieve a more comfortable relationship.

In this case, the patient's problems could be resolved by his talking things out with someone skilled in psychotherapy. When his troubles were approached in this way, Billy's memory complaints disappeared and his sleep patterns returned to normal. Moreover, he became much less anxious and fearful than he had been. His anxiety level decreased immediately after his problem was explained, and his first good night's sleep followed shortly thereafter. The noticeable improvement in his memory took almost two weeks, and it came as a very pleasant surprise to him.

Memory Defects in Depression

We all have life adjustment problems, of course, and from time to time each of us is susceptible to mild depression.

What we have to remember is that if we suddenly become forgetful, or if memory loss becomes a major concern to us, we should first try to discover if the real underlying problem is depression.

Depression affects the memory process in several different ways. Most important, it is often associated with hyperdistractibility; we just have too much on our minds. A depressed individual, even one with mild depression, is less able to focus attention and concentrate. Environmental impulses are thus much less likely to be formed into memory engrams in the brain, and even if engrams are formed, because information processing has been somewhat interfered with, they are defective. The neuropsychologist might call these defective engrams shallow memory traces. Because they are less permanent, the rate of forgetting is increased. In other words, their storage in the memory bank in any useful form is less likely.

Another defect in the memory mechanism which is common in depressed patients is that they are slow to retrieve specific memories. This can be true even though they often don't show any loss of memory at a more generalized level. Retrieving and reconstituting memories from their memory banks is a chore, although eventually they are able to dredge up the information they're searching for.

Depression, then, produces several defects in memory processing. Because of hyperdistractibility and lack of concentration it interferes with acquisition of new memories. It also interferes with retrieval from the memory bank and reconstitution, so that recall also becomes defective.

Some psychologists claim that memory impairment is not present in mild cases of depression, but this is certainly not my experience. For example, the experience of a long-time family friend, Clarence, demonstrates that mild and easily remedied depression can produce annoying changes in memory abilities.

I had known Clarence since the time both our families lived in the same city. He was an extremely bright and capable electrical engineer and certainly one of the nicest people I have ever known. After he left the air force he went to work for a Defense Department contractor, and about two years ago he retired to live in California.

He had always prided himself on his superior memory, but Clarence called me recently to say he was having great difficulty remembering the names of persons whose faces he was familiar with. He added, ominously, that the problem was getting worse.

I went over a number of possible factors — his daily activities, his diet, his challenges — and found one particular area that was disturbing him. His wife of many years, who was four or five years younger than he, also prided herself on her ability to remember names. They were walking together on a beach one day when they encountered an old acquaintance whose name Clarence could not remember. His wife, however, came up with the name immediately. Clarence gradually came to the conclusion that he was losing his memory when this same sequence was repeated several times over. This in turn precipitated a reactive depression that made his memory problem much worse.

I told Clarence it wasn't unusual for people as they grow older to have some difficulty recalling names, and that this was true even of persons with superior memories. Furthermore, I told him he sounded depressed, and he admitted it. He finally realized that the cause of his depression was that his wife seemed to have an easier time remembering names than he, which meant to him that he was failing. With this recognition and some dietary changes — the addition of B vitamins and lecithin in concentrated form — I told him to try again and see if things didn't improve.

Three or four weeks later I got a long distance telephone call from Clarence, who was bubbling over with enthusiasm.

He said that he and his wife had been walking in a shopping center when they encountered a couple they hadn't seen in years. His wife couldn't come up with the couple's names, but the names appeared in Clarence's mind like magic. While I was pleased that his depression had lifted and his memory abilities returned, I advised him to learn from his experience and not to put so much pressure on himself to remember names, especially in competition with his wife.

Severe Depression

More severe cases of depression produce more intense difficulties with memory. However, it is hard to correlate the degree of memory loss with the degree of depression exactly, partly because of the inexact criteria for gauging the intensity of the depressed state. Many psychologists and even psychiatrists feel that the suicidal patient suffers the most intense of the forms of depression. Here again, my experience says otherwise. There is a deeper depression that leaves the patient so apathetic that any meaningful behavior, including a suicide attempt, is almost impossible.

The most severely depressed patient is the one who has psychomotor retardation — an inability to plan for the future or even to move. Such patients will often lie in an almost mute state, unable to feed themselves or to wipe away the tears that well up in their eyes. They may have urinary retention, an inability to empty their bladders. They have a genuine loss of vital memory; testing patients in this state shows that almost all memory processing and intellectual abilities have been impeded. Because of their psychomotor retardation, it is difficult for them to carry out any complex behavior — including an attempt to commit suicide.

When treatment begins, whether it consists of drugs, electroshock treatment, or even surgery, and patients get better — their mood improves, they're able to feed themselves and take care of many of their own needs — at this point in the clinical course the danger of suicide becomes greater. Psychologists, psychiatrists, or other physicians managing these clinical cases must be aware of the potential for this devastating action and take appropriate preventive measures.

Ellen was such a patient. She had been treated by a Harvard psychiatrist for over twenty-five years for recurrent and severe depression. She repeatedly tried psychotherapy and group therapy and had successively taken the whole gamut of antidepressant medications known to physicians at the time. When none of these worked her psychiatrist, who was very conservative, reluctantly called in another specialist to administer electroshock treatments. These produced some transient memory loss, but also a temporary improvement in her depression.

Even with a full complement of medications, Ellen still required four more courses of electroshock treatments during the next ten years to reverse her steadily worsening depression. Because she was deteriorating and her psychiatrist didn't know what else to do, he called on me to operate on the limbic portion of her brain to try to alleviate her depression. When I first saw her she was lying in her bed staring at the ceiling, unable to wipe the tears from her cheeks, unable to urinate, unable to feed herself, unable to drink water, even when a straw was held to her lips.

I performed an operation in which a tiny electrode was inserted into a central area of her brain called the anterior nucleus of the thalamus. There were only two points out of thirty-six electrodes which, when stimulated, produced an exacerbation of anxiety and depression, and these points were destroyed by a tiny heat lesion generated by radio-frequency current.

After surgery, Ellen had a profound loss of recent memory, which lasted for six to eight weeks. When the memory loss began to disappear, however, it was obvious that her depression had substantially lifted. She was able to talk rationally with her psychiatrist, who was enthusiastic about her ability to take care of herself and plan for the future. Clinically she got better and better.

The day came when Ellen was allowed to shop by herself in a downtown department store. In the basement rest room of Filene's she took some poison she had carefully secreted in her handbag and committed suicide.

The effects of surgery had at first been encouraging. Ellen's mood and memory were greatly improved, and her psychomotor retardation was reversed — just the results we wanted from the operation. But surgical treatment contributed only a part, indeed a minor part, to Ellen's therapy. Unfortunately, Ellen's psychiatrist was deceived by the apparent clinical change in his patient. He did not realize that in spite of her remarkable improvement in mood she was still dangerously suicidal. This paradoxical therapeutic effect can be seen with medical as well as surgical therapies of depression. You should bring this fact to the attention of any physician treating a relative or friend of yours for depression. It could save a life. Just remember that an initial improvement in the mood of a severely depressed patient does not necessarily remove the danger of suicide.

Severe Depression in the Elderly

The loss of memory and other intellectual functions in severe depression can be quite profound. This is particularly true in patients who are over the age of fifty-five. Indeed, they may develop a clinical picture indistinguishable from that of the advanced stages of Alzheimer's disease.

Bridey, an eighty-two-year-old woman, had been in the Rose Manor Nursing Home for six years. She shared a room with a woman who had Alzheimer's disease, and the two behaved and acted very similarly. It was impossible to question her because she wouldn't respond appropriately or even obey simple commands. She would sit all day long, staring at the walls, and because she had developed cataracts in the lenses of both eyes what little visual information might have reached her brain was reduced substantially.

Bridey had also been somewhat hard of hearing in both ears for a number of years, so she could communicate only with the help of a hearing aid. In addition, the sensory monotony of the nursing home worsened her depression. She had the annoying habit of turning the clicker on her hearing aid off whenever anyone came around to visit her. This seemed to be the only purposeful thing she did do because she required assistance with most everything else, including feeding and bathroom functions.

In order to communicate with Bridey, I turned her hearing aid on and unwittingly increased the volume all the way up, producing a high-pitched, piercing sound. She roused from her lethargy and turned the hearing aid off, but in doing so said quite clearly, "Stop that racket. Can't you leave me alone?" This fragment of speech was so unlike any response she had ever exhibited — in other examinations, in her clinical history, and in what was thought to be her clinical state as an end-stage Alzheimer's patient with complete memory loss — that I immediately began various treatments for depression.

Over a period of several weeks the treatments with an antidepressant called Prozac became more and more effective. This drug does not have some of the side effects of other antidepressants, but the therapist has to be very patient in using it because it can take up to a couple of months for the effects of the drug to become clinically apparent.* As Bridey became more talkative and more open to therapy, her geri-

*Prozac may have the paradoxical effect of not averting suicide attempts in a small number of depressed patients whose energy level is improved by the drug.

atric psychiatrist discovered the reasons for her depressed state.

The psychiatrist found that Bridey, like many elderly patients who are forced to live in nursing homes, had wanted to conserve her assets for her children. She had therefore transferred those assets to them, leaving herself penniless and a candidate for Medicaid. Sadly, however, once her children had control of her assets they disappeared from her life, leaving her alone, disillusioned, and disappointed in a constricting world in which environmental stimuli were monotonous and uninspiring. She was in a state of partial sensory deprivation compounded by feelings of loss and abandonment by her own children. This was especially disturbing to her because she had been quite close to her children. She had been their sole support when they were growing up, after her alcoholic husband had abandoned the family early in her marriage and was never heard from again.

Bridey's children, a son and a daughter in their forties, each had their own families and interests. The sudden gift of money to them from their mother, who had been a prudent saver and a wise investor, had temporarily diverted them from their family obligations. When they did come to see Bridey they found her in an obviously demented state with very poor memory functions, so they decided there wasn't anything more they could do. But they became much more attentive when they learned the real facts of the case, which helped ensure that their mother would not again slip into a profound depression — what is often called the pseudodementia of depression.

While it certainly helped Bridey, Prozac is not the only effective antidepressant. A number of other agents are available, each acting on different aspects of brain chemistry. Some of these agents, however, although they are potent antidepressants, also interfere with the brain's use of acetylcholine, a neurotransmitter associated with the memory process. It is thus possible for an antidepressant to relieve depression and at the same time make memory loss worse. I therefore always urge treating psychiatrists or physicians to be aware of this potential and adjust dosage and change drugs if it is clinically necessary.

Later I discuss some of the more widely used antidepressants and their side effects. Here, however, I want to make you aware of what may be an important new treatment in reversing depression and memory loss: a therapy called transcranial electrical brain stimulation (which is *not* the same as electroshock or electroconvulsive therapy). I firmly believe this therapy will prove effective in treating a great number of depressed patients during the next decade and reduce their need for medication. It too will be examined more fully in subsequent chapters.

Stress, Depression, and Memory Loss

At times in life everyone experiences stressful situations: illness, financial difficulties, even physical danger. The initial response to stress is usually heightened awareness and increased vigilance. But if the stress continues for a long period of time, depression sets in. Everything seems to be closing in on the person, there don't seem to be any options, and a depressed mood almost inevitably results.

As we've seen already, depression is frequently associated with hyperdistractibility, decreased attention span, and decreased concentration, which causes new memories to be improperly encoded in the limbic brain and often makes the retrieval of remote memories from the memory bank slow and inefficient. Another response to severe stress related to depression is that the depressed brain is susceptible to being overwhelmed by shocking events. The combination of depression and severe stress can produce a dramatic loss of memory in what is known as transient global amnesia.

Transient Global Amnesia

Nathan, fifty-two, was a hard-driving businessman with political ambitions. When the incumbent in the district race for state senator dropped out because of ill health, Nathan took the plunge and used his own resources to enter the contest.

Nathan's position of strength, power, and experience in his business dealings gave him the assurance to be successful. In politics, however, his experience was nil. He therefore hired a campaign manager, Phil, who was equally hard-driving and extremely arrogant. Phil took over not only Nathan's campaign but also his life, ordering Nathan's routine and overseeing every facet of his activities. As the relationship became more and more irritating to Nathan, a series of explosive confrontations erupted between Nathan and Phil. Phil was used to such conflicts, but Nathan, who had been accustomed to the more serene atmosphere of commerce, was not. Nathan became very depressed.

Late one morning he decided he'd had enough and called Phil to sever the relationship. A vitriolic shouting match ensued between the two of them which could be heard all over Nathan's house. His wife noticed he had a confused look on his face when he hung up the telephone, but when she questioned him he said he didn't remember any phone conversation. In fact, he had difficulty remembering the layout of his own house. He didn't know the month or year, and he had no recollection of having entered a political campaign.

Nathan entered a state of complete bewilderment. His loss of memory extended back to events that had occurred five to six months before the explosive telephone conversation with Phil. He couldn't remember from one minute to the next what happened after the call. His wife, panic-stricken, called a doctor for an immediate appointment. I was brought in shortly afterward as a consulting neurologist.

At first I didn't know what to make of Nathan, but as I

started to examine him some of his memory faculties slowly but definitely began to return. At the end of two hours, much of his memory had been restored, except that he still had a loss of recent and ongoing memory. He had no recollection of the telephone conversation itself, but he did remember that he was a political candidate and what had happened the previous day.

I thought Nathan might have had a seizure — that perhaps he had been on some tranquilizing medication and had had it withdrawn suddenly. But this was not the case. Blood tests were normal; his neurological examination showed nothing unusual, and a CAT scan of his brain revealed no abnormalities. Furthermore, a computerized brain wave test, which ought to have shown some abnormal slowing if Nathan was in the recovery stages of an epileptic seizure, was absolutely normal.

What was wrong with Nathan? He had a condition known as transient global amnesia, a relatively benign loss of memory in that most persons who experience it recover almost completely and rarely have a recurrence of the problem. What causes it? Some researchers attribute transient global amnesia to a shower of tiny strokes in the memory centers deep in the brain, but no strong evidence supports this theory, and certainly there was no evidence of a stroke in Nathan's case. There was also no sign of a seizure or of any head injury. Nathan had a history of migraine attacks earlier in his life, but he hadn't had one for a long time.

Some neurologists think that transient global amnesia is a rare manifestation of migraine. Perhaps a better explanation of Nathan's case is that so much accumulated stress simply overloaded his neural circuits, which were already sensitized by depression. In fact, it is not uncommon that a history of great and sometimes overwhelming stress just precedes an attack of transient global amnesia.

I believe that stress, particularly overwhelming stress, in a patient who is already depressed may produce severe transient memory loss. The moral of Nathan's experience is not that you should completely avoid all stress, but that your lifestyle should include stress-relieving exercises, which also help dissolve some forms of reactive depression (that is, depression resulting as a reaction to some event).

Some physicians view transient global amnesia as a simply psychological response to environmental stress. I disagree with this notion. The brains of patients I've seen with this disorder have been made more susceptible to severe stress by depression. The result of overwhelming stress on a depressed individual is a brain dysfunction that, although environmental or psychological in its origin, temporarily results in organic malfunction — that is, focal or isolated suppression of brain activity, in this case memory. Fortunately, the condition is transient. Patients almost always recover, and recurrence of the problem is rare.

Vital Memory Points to Remember

1. Depression is the most common, and most easily misdiagnosed, reversible cause of memory loss.
2. There are different kinds of depression, all of which cause different degrees of memory loss and each of which requires different kinds of treatment (e.g., psychotherapy for life adjustment problems and medication for neurochemical imbalance).
3. Alcohol may induce a brief euphoria, but it also makes any kind of depression worse.
4. Depression makes one less able to focus attention and concentration and slows memory retrieval.
5. Overwhelming stress may produce severe transient memory loss in persons whose brains have already been incapacitated by depression.
6. Almost all kinds of memory loss associated with depression can be reversed.

64

6

Alcoholism, Brain Poisoning, and Memory Loss

Do you drink an alcoholic beverage every day? Has anyone ever told you that you drink too much? Do you have problems remembering things that are important to you? Have you ever had gaps in your memory, especially after drinking heavily — times that you can't seem to remember what went on, whether for a few hours or even days? Do you find that your memory isn't as sharp now as it was six months or a year ago? If you answered yes to any of these questions, the amount of alcohol you're drinking may be affecting your memory.

This is not to say that anyone who has an occasional (that is, once a month) glass of wine or other alcoholic drink will be irrevocably brain-damaged. But especially if your diet is insufficient or poorly balanced, if you drink every day and feel that your memory abilities are slipping, there are a few facts you need to know. First and foremost, alcohol is a poison.

Alcohol Poisoning
Alcohol poisons the brain and uniformly depresses brain function. The first area of the brain to be affected by alcohol is the limbic, or emotional area of the brain. This was

65

originally shown by J. C. Lee, a Canadian scientist who studied the breakdown of the blood-brain barrier in experimental animals after intravascular administration of various amounts of alcohol.

Under ordinary circumstances the blood-brain barrier is a barrier around the capillaries in the brain which prevents unwanted substances from getting into brain cells. But if something disrupts its ability to block substances from entering brain cells, dramatic things can happen in the brain, such as excessive accumulation of ions and chemicals around the cells. Normally the blood-brain barrier keeps ions and chemicals at proper proportions and concentrations for healthy brain function. Calcium ions, for example, are a normal component of the nerve cell environment, but if the blood-brain barrier ceases to operate effectively the consequent buildup of calcium ions can cause brain cell death.

The blood-brain barrier can be broken down by such traumas as brain injury, hemorrhage, tumors, infection, and extreme alteration of the ratio of oxygen to carbon dioxide in the blood that reaches the brain. Alcohol in the blood stream also breaks down the barrier. Significant amounts break down the barrier throughout the entire brain; small amounts break it down only in the limbic brain — the inner parts of the temporal lobes, known as the hippocampus and the amygdala, and the midline parts of the brain, the thalamus and hypothalamus.

One effect of this poisoning of the limbic brain is that the inhibitory restraints that generally govern social conduct and interpersonal relationships are lifted. You have only to stand outside the door of a room where a cocktail party is in progress to measure this breakdown of the blood-brain barrier and the initial poisoning of the emotional brain in the people who are drinking inside. You can hear it. As the limbic brains of more and more of the participants are poisoned, voices become louder and more shrill and the noise of the party increases to a crescendo. After a while, when people's brains become more thoroughly poisoned, the depressing effects of alcohol become apparent and the party goers become sleepy. If they drink enough, they can even become unconscious.

During the initial phase of brain poisoning, when the inhibitory centers are depressed, persons consuming alcohol do not feel that they have lost intellectual ability. Many people feel slightly elated and grossly overestimate their abilities, including their faculty of memory as well as other intellectual capacities. There may be a very short-term effect initially which makes it appear to individuals that they're able to concentrate better than they could before they began drinking. They often feel they can focus attention on whatever they're doing without the distractions from the outside world which normally worry them or the difficulties stemming from the past which make them less able to function. But this brief period of elation, which is associated with a lack of concern for real-world problems and of capacity for reality testing, quickly passes into a state of general unconcern in which all phases of the memory process are depressed.

Alcohol Poisoning and Memory Loss

Chronic alcohol abuse can produce memory loss in different ways. As people drink, the focusing of attention becomes more difficult, acquisition of new information can be retarded, the memory traces stored are more shallow, and the rate of forgetting of new memories is increased. In addition, the retrieval of memories from the memory bank is also slowed down, and accompanying this increased retrieval time is greater difficulty reconstituting memories. All intellectual functions are diminished. Finally, new memories are simply not elaborated. Many people who drink steadily over a period of hours or days are left with blank spots in their memories in place of a record of what happened during the period of their intoxication — the so-called Lost Weekend.

Memory deficits in people who consume large amounts of alcohol are often difficult to ascribe to one cause to the exclusion of others. While it is true that people drinking alcohol are poisoning their brains, other factors may enter the clinical picture, making the precise cause of memory loss difficult to define. Nutritional deficiencies, for example, are common among persons who consume large amounts of alcohol (perhaps 6 percent of the adult population; 10 percent of those who drink alcohol can be classified as alcohol abusers or alcoholics). Certain B vitamins are often lacking in the diets of alcohol abusers, especially vitamin B-1, or thiamine. Thiamine deficiency is associated with a disease called Korsakoff's psychosis, which produces a memory loss and can be corrected only if the thiamine and vitamins B-5 and B-6 are taken in sufficient quantities to saturate the tissue before permanent brain damage occurs.

Repeated or chronic use of alcohol in intoxicating quantities is also associated with brain injury because drunken people tend to fall down and get into accidents. Closed-head injuries often damage the under surface of the frontal lobes and the anterior parts of the temporal lobes, the area of the brain where the acquisition of new memories occurs.

During the withdrawal stage, alcoholism can bring on epileptic seizures, another cause of memory loss since seizures often begin in the inner part of the temporal lobes in the centers closely related to the acquisition of new memories. Alcoholic seizure, or a "rum fit," is one of the most frequently cited reasons for patients' being admitted to city hospitals.

All of these factors may operate in patients who take in large amounts of alcohol. In some people who are very susceptible, even small amounts of alcohol can have the same effects. For example, a person with any kind of brain injury or brain tumor may set off a train of epileptic seizures with only one or two drinks. My advice to patients with brain tumors, strokes, or injuries is not to drink at all.

Another aspect of the effects of drinking is that many persons who abuse alcohol do so in a vain effort to treat underlying depression. The depression has already reduced certain memory abilities, and of course the use of the alcohol only exacerbates tendencies toward impaired memory function.

Some physicians and brain researchers believe that the effects of alcohol on the brain are really the result of vitamin deficiencies, brain injury, or epileptic seizures related to the use of alcohol. My own experience, however, does not bear this out. Alcohol poisoning by itself, even in healthy persons who have normal diets, produces a decrease in brain function and changes in the structure of the brain. Alterations in the soft tissue of the brain can easily be seen on CAT scans, which reveal a falling away or diminution of some tissues deep inside the brain with a corresponding expansion of spinal fluid into the vacated spaces. These spaces, or lateral ventricles, become very large at times but will often shrink when the alcoholic patient stops drinking.

Alcohol Abuse and Loss of Vital Memory

Chronic alcohol abuse can also produce a loss of intellectual faculties, including a loss of vital memory. The following case may seem like an extreme example, but in many ways it illustrates how alcohol can impair vital memory; in fact, the case of Kenny, one of our patients, was typical of this syndrome.

Before I saw Kenny he had been drinking excessively for years, to the point that he had difficulty even in performing the everyday activities of life. Unless he had the supervision of his wife, his behavior was so unpredictable that his own safety was threatened. Walking in Boston, for example, he would step out into a flow of fast-moving traffic. He didn't recognize his peril in such circumstances, even when he was comparatively sober. In other words, Kenny had lost vital memory about the danger of getting in the way of fast-moving cars; he had lost essential parts of his memory which would keep him out of harm's way.

You may think that there was something peculiar about Kenny — that he didn't eat well or had always been lazy. But before he started drinking too much Kenny had had a good job, and his wife was devoted to him. Even after his heavy drinking began, his wife made sure he ate nutritious meals. Nevertheless, Kenny developed a swelling of the fluid-filled spaces in his brain, with shrinkage of deep tissues. The swellings indicated structural brain damage caused by excessive alcohol intake.

My impression that chronic alcohol abuse causes deteriorating brain function has been confirmed by psychologists like Nelson Butters and his associates. Butters found that alcoholics with adequate nutrition who abstained from all alcoholic beverages still performed well below average in certain learning tasks requiring good recent-memory function. Alcoholics suffering a decrease in their short-term verbal memory were less able to recognize famous faces and did less well than normal controls on tests of recall, a function that dropped off still further among older alcoholic subjects.

Although chronic alcoholics scored substantially lower than normal controls, they still did better than Korsakoff's patients, who have the added problem of vitamin B-1 deficiency. This fact indicates to me that even though thiamine deficiency interrupts memory functions, particularly recent memory, much more powerfully than chronic alcoholism alone, the brain poisoning caused by long-term alcohol abuse plays a role in persistent and progressive memory loss, even after the patient has stopped drinking.

Myths of Alcohol Consumption

No one is immune to the effects of alcohol, and no one is protected from its dangerous side effects. The case history of Kenny may lead you to think that you're in trouble only if you're an alcohol abuser with severely impaired brain function. But that's not true. In one experiment, for example, we tested the neurological function of clergymen who drank frequently but in most other ways were performing normally. Because of their institutional setting these persons' nutrition was excellent, and because of their calling they had superior intellectual ability. Even so, our subjects exhibited decreases in mental function and some aspects of memory. Many of them, who had regularly consumed moderate amounts of alcohol, showed a loss of tissue in the medial part of the frontal lobes, resulting in a widening of the fissure between the two cerebral hemispheres and a decrease in brain tissue in the inner part of the frontal lobes. Long-term alcohol use, we thus concluded, even by well-nourished individuals, produces structural changes in the brain.

The most important fact you should know about alcohol is that it is a brain poison; it disturbs normal brain function. People use it, as they have for millennia, as a shield from the harsh realities of everyday existence. The occasional person, such as Winston Churchill, may abuse alcohol and still be very productive. But for every person who is so fortunate as to escape the long-term results of alcohol poisoning, there are thousands of others who suffer its deleterious effects. Alexander the Great, whose epileptic seizures were probably exacerbated by his abuse of alcohol, and whose premature death at age thirty-three was probably related to his immoderate drinking, is a well-documented historical example.

But without enumerating the famous or infamous persons whose lives were destroyed by alcohol, I want to stress that the average individual who poisons his or her brain with alcohol is less able to solve the problems one encounters from day to day in our competitive and complex society. Memory impairment by brain poisoning makes us less prepared and less resourceful in responding to the challenges of our world.

My own view is that for optimal brain function the intake

71

of alcohol should be zero. I base my opinion on data recorded during Prohibition, when as a nation we tried the social experiment of trying to eliminate all alcohol consumption. The experiment failed because of the corruption and greed of the public officials responsible for managing it. Nevertheless, Prohibition was a conspicuous medical success. The years during which the manufacture and sale of alcohol were outlawed in the United States saw a great reduction in deaths from cirrhosis of the liver and an even more striking decrease in the number of admissions to state mental hospitals for alcohol-related psychosis. We'll undoubtedly never return to prohibition in this country, but the data prove conclusively that reduced alcohol consumption benefits health.

I am always asked about those over fifty who take a drink to improve digestion. Alcohol does stimulate the stomach's secretion of hydrochloric acid (which is why it is bad for people with ulcers). But other gastric stimulants for persons whose secretion of hydrochloric acid is deficient can be prescribed by a physician once such a diagnosis has been confirmed.

Finally, there is the question of the celebratory glass of wine taken once a month or once a week. How much harm will a single glass of wine or can of beer do to the brain? The answer is that we don't know. If a person seldom drinks, having a glass of wine or beer at parties perhaps four or five times a year, the chances are that such a small level of consumption will have a negligible effect. Drinking beer or wine every day, however, is potentially harmful to brain cells. And as an individual progresses from beer or wine to whiskey or cocktails, the effects become definitely harmful.

The common denominator is not what kind of alcoholic beverage is drunk but how much alcohol is getting to the brain. On average, heavier people tolerate alcohol better than thin people and men better than women. Also, some individuals have more protective enzymes to detoxify alcohol than

72

others. Once alcohol gets to the brain in sufficient concentrations, however, it is poisonous. The important issues are the intensity of the poison, the duration of its effects, and how healthy one's brain is to begin with. Even drinking a lot of beer can severely poison your brain, although the proportion of alcohol in each glass is small.

The choice is yours to make. Your brain is the most precious organ in your body. It needs the utmost protection — especially from brain poisons. All of us often balance, whether consciously or not, the pleasure a particular behavior gives us against the risks. When you drink you know about the pleasure, but you may think that the only risk you face is a hangover. Unfortunately, continual use of alcohol may have long-term adverse consequences on your memory and thought processes, consequences that are not completely reversible even when you stop drinking. The sad fact is that you may not even be aware of your loss until some novel challenge or emergency arises which requires you to make the nice judgment or the right choice that your brain is no longer capable of making. In other words, you may not realize how much damage you've done until it's too late to fix it.

If you feel that you must have alcohol every day, you may have to change your lifestyle, such as by cutting out the nightly cocktail or beer you have while watching television, or not having that glass of wine at every social gathering you attend. It may ultimately mean a reevaluation of the balance between pleasure and pain. If you're in doubt as to where you stand, perhaps you should have a detailed neuropsychological test performed to see if you are slipping mentally and therefore need to reduce or eliminate alcohol from your diet.

Vital Memory Points to Remember
1. Alcohol is related to 10 percent of all deaths in the United States each year.

2. Alcohol is a tissue poison that acts on the limbic area of the brain.
3. Even small amounts of alcohol break down the blood-brain barrier.
4. Joining an organization such as Alcoholics Anonymous is a good first step in helping you control a drinking problem.

7

The Effects of Stimulants, Depressants, and Drugs That Produce Hallucinations on Memory and Intelligence

MOST OF US during our lives experiment with drugs by drinking alcohol or using coffee, tea, or tobacco. Some of us experiment with marijuana, cocaine, speed, or even heroin. While I don't equate the use of coffee or tobacco with that of speed or heroin, all these agents have something in common: they affect and even poison the limbic portion of our brains. If they didn't have such an effect hardly anyone would use them. And, of course, our memory functions are centered in the limbic brain and are influenced in one way or another by all of these drugs.

Some people get hooked on street drugs quite innocently. Some heroin abusers began as patients with chronic pain who were given long-term medical treatment with narcotics. Some people who abuse speed were prescribed diet pills by their physicians which contained a speedlike component, and they became hooked on amphetamines. The chronic use of these drugs not only made them amphetamine-dependent but also produced personality changes, including mood disturbances and paranoia. Many of these persons develop cross dependencies on other street drugs and alcohol as well.

The point is that all street drugs, when used frequently over a long period of time, have bad effects on the brain, including depression, craving for drugs, reduced memory and intellectual abilities, and epileptic seizures. Also, these effects may linger after drug use has been discontinued and crop up months and even years later, which indicates the long-term deleterious effects of many of these agents.

Stimulants

In addition to patients who inadvertently became hooked on amphetamines by taking diet pills, I've met many people in my medical practice who take stimulants to "improve" thinking and memory or just to feel better and be more energetic. They get an initial lift in feeling and mental prowess, but it doesn't last. And using amphetamines and speed over and over produces just the opposite of the results they wanted. This happened to Jerry, who should have known better because he was a medical student.

Jerry was twenty-five years old, had an attractive smile, and was quite popular. But although I considered him to be a bright young man, I knew he thought of himself as an underachiever. That's because Jerry tested very low on standard intelligence tests, and his scores on the college aptitude boards were so inferior that he was not able to gain admission to a regular college but had to go to a remedial one until he showed he could keep up the quality of work necessary in college studies.

That he did well enough not only to graduate from college but also to be admitted to medical school was a surprise to both him and his parents. But he never believed he had accomplished this on his own. He thought his performance in medical school depended on his use of a chemical stimulant, an amphetamine-like drug that fell in the category of street drugs known as speed.

In small amounts this drug did speed up his mental processes, allowing him to focus more intensely on the subjects he was studying and to retain the information well enough to pass tests. But then he forgot everything he had learned very quickly and had to start all over again for the next examination.

Over a period of time Jerry found that he couldn't achieve the same scholastic results with the small amount of stimulant he had been using, and so of course he increased the dose. With the increased dose, however, he was distressed to find that his powers of concentration didn't improve, but got worse. He became agitated and hyperdistractible, he couldn't concentrate, and he wasn't able to focus his attention with enough intensity to retain the material he had to learn to pass his examinations. As a result, his grades began to fall off. His performance as a student deteriorated to the point that he was failing some of his courses and just barely passing others. Jerry also began to undergo personality changes, becoming rather suspicious and at times aggressive.

The sad part of Jerry's story is that he did have the ability to be a satisfactory student without using mind-altering drugs. This realization grew on him only very slowly, and at great personal cost. In the interim, Jerry learned with much anguish his lesson about the addictive nature of stimulants.

The story has a happy ending: Jerry finally got himself off drugs and graduated from medical school — but just barely. He went on to pass his medical boards and became a competent physician.

The effects that stimulants had on Jerry are not unusual. The initial dose, particularly if it is small, will often enhance memory function and increase concentration; it also brings about some elevation of mood, which also helps in focusing attention. As the dose is increased, however, the three elements of memory, acquisition, storage, and retrieval, begin to deteriorate, and performance, particularly with regard to new learning, is diminished.

Ingesting excessive amounts of these medications can produce an acute confusional state marked by disorientation and

even hallucinations. Meaningful memory testing is often impossible in these circumstances. Some neurological purists
doubt that memory loss occurs in this state because significant testing can't be done. My view, however, is that vital
memory is always lost in confusional states characterized by
disorientation. In other words, if you don't know where or
who you are or what the year or season is, your vital memory
is seriously impaired.

Repeated use of stimulants only enhances their negative
effects. The elevation of mood proceeds too far, to hyperexcit-
ability, which in turn leads to distraction, not concentration,
and consequent difficulty in acquiring new information for
storage in the memory bank.

Special considerations must be applied in the self-adminis-
tration of various illegal stimulants because they are sometimes used to reverse the symptoms of underlying depression. The results are uniformly disappointing, and sometimes
dangerous.

Cocaine is often used for this purpose, especially if the
depression is of the bipolar variety called manic-depressive
illness. All too often the euphoria produced by a dose of
cocaine is followed by a depression that is much worse than
the original one. The anxiety and hyperactivity associated
with cocaine effects, however, may not disappear even when
the rebound depression is full-blown. Of course the effects
on every aspect of memory, concentration, and new learning
are devastating. As with amphetamines, cocaine can also lead
to states of increased suspiciousness and even paranoid de-
lusions.

Some cocaine users go on to become aggressive and even
dangerous in initiating unprovoked attack behavior. Their
memories are selectively and sometimes randomly inhibited
during these episodes, and they may not remember their actions afterward. Cocaine can also provoke epileptic seizures or
start the kindling of epileptic seizures in the emotional brain.

Such abnormal electrical activity is so close to the memory circuits that it may severely disrupt memory function.

The stimulant drugs that are very closely related to amphetamines, such as methylamphetamine, can cause lasting disturbances in brain function in terms of decreasing memory abilities. Almost all the stimulant-type drugs are dangerous as far as memory and brain integrity are concerned, both functionally and structurally. Related compounds like Ritalin, however, are used therapeutically in hyperactive children with minimal brain damage and have the paradoxical effect of calming them down and improving their ability to retain new information. But even Ritalin has unwanted effects on the brains of normal people, and a substantial amount of medical controversy still swirls around the use of this agent.

Coffee, Tea, and Tobacco

Coffee, tea, and tobacco are the most common brain stimulants, although of a much milder sort. The use of tobacco has the most ominous health effects of the three not only because of the carcinogenic potential of tars and nicotine and their action in provoking abnormalities in the lungs, blood vessels, and heart but also because nicotine is intensely addictive.

Many people who drink coffee think that it helps them concentrate. A recent study of the effects of caffeine on healthy college students, however, showed only an insignificant influence on learning and memory performance. A small dose of caffeine decreased boredom and relaxation and increased certain subjective moods such as anxiety, tenseness, and nervousness. Many moderate to frequent users of coffee felt that it helped their recall. In any case, the actual effect of coffee on memory is difficult to assess because the effect is so small.

At a radio station where I was to speak I was recently approached by a young woman employee of the station who

79

asked, in a quiet voice so no one else could hear, whether she could improve her memory and recall for a major examination by drinking a lot of coffee or taking caffeine pills. It was an important test, one that she was concerned about doing well on, and she had heard that drinking coffee while studying and taking the test would improve her performance. I explained that caffeine might confer a minor benefit in that perhaps her attention span would improve, but that she ran the risk of becoming even more agitated, which would ultimately cancel any benefits of better concentration. As unpatronizingly as I could, I gave her my best advice: to study as much as possible and get a good night's sleep before the exam.

Depressants

Sedative drugs, including alcohol, have a marked effect in depressing memory, and the effects are dose-dependent. The higher the blood level of the agent used, the more likely one is to impair all phases of memory function. These agents were originally used medically to combat epileptic seizures. Many years ago, bromides were the drug of choice, but they had so many severe side effects that they were supplanted by the barbiturates. While barbiturates did control some epileptic seizures and the anxiety that surrounded them, they also produced a strong sedative effect. It was once not uncommon, before the advent of Dilantin, to see epileptic patients walk around looking like zombies, barely able to keep their eyes open. Of course, memory function was terribly impaired in this group of patients. Barbiturates were also widely prescribed as sleeping pills and tranquilizers, but the word *sedative* was substituted for *tranquilizer*.

More recently the barbiturates have been supplanted by the so-called minor tranquilizers. Although Valium has a limited use in controlling seizures, this and other agents are chiefly prescribed for their sedative effects. I'm speaking of not only Valium but such drugs as Ativan, Librium, Serax, Xanax, and Atarax. I don't mean to suggest that these agents don't have a place in medicine; they do. Xanax in particular is very useful in treating a certain kind of panic disorder. What I do know is that their role in medicine should be much more circumscribed than is now the case.

Millions of Americans take these drugs, even though many patients don't need them. Almost all of these patients have a degree of impaired memory as a result (if you measure memory abilities after the administration of the drugs and compare them with memory abilities before the drugs were started). Most of these drugs produce substantial memory impairment after the first day of administration. In some cases the impairment may be so severe that whole episodes of the patient's life are forgotten. In some ways this pattern resembles the Lost Weekend syndrome caused by imbibing large amounts of alcohol, which also depresses brain function.

Elderly persons are often given these tranquilizers to quiet their anxieties, and they are generally more susceptible to their poisonous effects on their memories. Reducing dosage can be therapeutic.

Hallucinogens

Hallucinogenic drugs are taken for no other purpose than to produce hallucinations or visions in the brains of people using them. Some hallucinogenic drugs are synthesized in the laboratory, and the chemist can combine hallucinogens with stimulants to tailor-make a drug to the abuser's wishes, producing a so-called designer drug.

One of the more strikingly effective hallucinogens is LSD-25. This drug, derived from the ergot fungus, was the outcome of the twenty-fifth experiment conducted with the fungus by a Swiss chemist, Dr. A. Hofman. It produces the vivid hallucinations and distortions of time characteristic of all these agents.

81

One of my psychiatric colleagues at the Massachusetts General Hospital was called on to treat several graduate students in theoretical mathematics at the Massachusetts Institute of Technology who, after experimenting with LSD, suffered recurring hallucinations after they stopped using the drug. Through prolonged treatment he was able to relieve their immediate symptoms, but he noted over the long term that their intellectual abilities and their memories had deteriorated. These were brilliant, productive people before they started their experimentation with drugs, and they were still smart even after the effects of the drug had worn off. But the use of LSD had decreased their intelligence and their memory abilities slightly yet permanently. Their creative abilities were also somewhat diminished, and many realized they were no longer able to contribute new ideas in their field. The diminution in their abilities was caused by the concentration of this chemical agent in the inner part of the emotional brain, a part called the hippocampus, which produced a deterioration in cells also serving in the memory circuitry. Similar drugs, like PCPs and Angel Dust, do the same thing and often cause epileptic seizures.

One of the most commonly abused hallucinogens in the United States is marijuana. There has been a lot of controversy over whether this agent has deleterious effects on the brain. Extensive studies of the effects of marijuana leave no question that it impairs learning and the retention of new information. In other words, its continued use does undermine memory.

Whether memory loss stemming from marijuana use is permanent or not is difficult to assess because we do not have the necessary psychological evaluations of chronic users of marijuana before they began smoking marijuana, so it is impossible to determine how much their intellectual abilities may have declined after using the drug. It is known, however, that smoking a single marijuana cigarette affects the brain, particularly in slowing reaction times. Of course marijuana, like other drugs — depressants (including tranquilizers), alcohol, stimulants, and hallucinogens — is taken because of its effect on the brain. Even very mild drugs are essentially brain toxins whose effects, even in low doses, result from an alteration or poisoning of brain function.

The central question is how much brain poisoning we can tolerate, and whether the poisoning is worth the feelings we get from having our inhibitions dampened or our moods elevated. Each person must answer this question for himself, but everyone should at least be aware of the harmful effects of these agents in suppressing memory and depressing brain function.

If you want to get off street drugs but can't do it by yourself, you should seek medical help from an addiction program near you. There is often a transference between drug abuse and alcohol abuse, so programs like Alcoholics Anonymous can also be helpful for some patients with drug problems. Don't be reluctant to ask for help, because kicking a drug habit can almost never be accomplished alone.

Vital Memory Points to Remember

1. The repeated use of stimulants tends to diminish memory abilities and capacity for new learning.
2. Cocaine use can cause memory impairment.
3. The actual effect of coffee drinking on memory is hard to assess because the effect is so small.
4. Almost all drugs that alter normal brain function will produce some degree of memory impairment if taken in sufficient quantities over a long enough period of time.

8

Prescription Medications That Cause Memory Loss

ARE YOU TAKING some kind of medication prescribed by your doctor which you've been on for a long time? Has your dose been changed recently, or have you been given a new medicine, one that you weren't on before? If so, have you noticed any change in your intelligence, memory, or mood since you started the new medicine or changed the amount of your old medicine? Or has there been any recent change in your memory, mood, or mental abilities, even though you haven't started on a new medicine or dosage? This happened to Henry, whose mental changes were related to the doctor-prescribed medicine he was taking.

Henry was a sixty-seven-year-old patient of mine who had severe intermittent abdominal pain. For thirty years he went from one physician to another and had a number of thorough examinations, including special x-ray tests, all of which failed to disclose the reason for his problem. He was finally diagnosed as having spastic bowel syndrome and was put on daily doses of phenobarbital and belladonna. Sometimes these medications worked and sometimes they didn't, but Henry kept taking them for months, and eventually years.

About nine months before I saw him he had begun to become more forgetful, generally duller, and less intellectually reactive to his wife and family. They thought he must be getting Alzheimer's disease, but our tests didn't indicate any specific problems in his brain except for some changes in his brain wave test which showed difficulty in brain metabolism.

When we examined the medications Henry had been taking, his wife assured me that he had been taking the same dose of each for many years. I was sure that the medications were the villains in causing his memory loss. Belladonna interferes with the brain's use of acetylcholine, the neurotransmitter related to the memory circuits in the inner part of the temporal lobes, whereas phenobarbital is long-acting and its effect tends to accumulate in the central nervous system. I didn't want simply to stop the medications, however, since a patient who has been on phenobarbital for a long time and suddenly stops taking it is very apt to have epileptic seizures.

What I did was gradually reduce the dosages of the medications. Within a few days, the lowered blood level of these drugs resulted in improvement in both Henry's memory and his intellectual function. After three weeks, by then on much-reduced doses, Henry was back to normal functioning and still free of pain.

The lesson to be learned from this case, and many similar ones, is that it isn't always necessary to discontinue someone's medication even though it may be directly related to their symptoms of impaired mental function and memory loss. Henry needed help for his abdominal pain, but that help had to be balanced with the consequences of consuming the medications. Sometimes just reducing the dosage of medication is enough to restore a patient's normal mental function.

One always has to stay alert to this need for balancing. Someone can take a medication at the same dosage for a long period of time without having any noticeable effects on the brain or brain function. Suddenly, when abrupt changes in lifestyle or in the inner chemistry and metabolism of the body (whether or not related to age) occur, the person can no longer tolerate the same dose of medication.

This finding is not unusual, and physicians should be aware of it, although sometimes they aren't. It is true for people of all ages but especially for the elderly, whose bodies can be slower in detoxifying or eliminating medications. Also, as we grow older we have fewer brain cells, and even if these cells function more efficiently, they are more susceptible to brain poisoning because there is less brain reserve. It is more difficult for an older person with fewer brain cells to recover from a serious brain insult, whether caused by brain injury or brain poisoning, than it is for a child, for example, who has many more brain cells.

Doctors certainly know that infants, children, and adults require different dosage schedules of medications. What they often fail to realize is that people over the age of fifty-five, and particularly over sixty, should follow a reduced dosage schedule. And of course, the older people get, the more susceptible they become to side effects from what might have been well-tolerated dosages of medications they took at a younger age, whether the drugs affected the brain or not.

You will notice that I have been focusing on the memory or intellectual changes that follow the use of a new drug or a change in dosage of one of the medicines you are currently taking. Drugs can produce many other kinds of changes, from sleep disturbances to dry mouth or itching. If you have any of these symptoms, it should be called to the attention of your doctor, but I have not discussed such symptoms in detail because they may not be related to your memory problems.

Every drug known to man has dose-dependent side effects or toxic consequences. A drug's side effects are usually listed by the manufacturer in a statement enclosed in the package. I urge you to read these statements. Unfortunately, many drug companies do not include the adverse effects of their com-

TABLE 1   **Potentially Toxic or Poisonous Prescription Drugs That Commonly Produce Problems with Memory or Intelligence**

Psychiatric Drugs	Drugs Used in General Medicine
Barbiturates	Digitalis preparations
Bromides	Analgesics
Benzodiazepams	Antihypertensives (especially beta blockers)
Phenothiazines	Antidiabetic agents
Haloperidol	Cimetidine
Lithium	Methyldopa
Antidepressants	Inderal
	Reserpine
	Symmetrel
	Drugs with anticholinergic actions (seasickness pills)
	Antihistamines
	Eye drops for glaucoma

Source: Dr. Thomas D. Sabin, Boston City Hospital.

pounds on brain function and memory, an omission I would like to see corrected.

Table 1 is a partial list of drugs that can alter memory and intellectual functions. In addition, certain combinations of drugs — Mellaril and lithium, for example, or haloperidol and methyldopa — are likely to produce confusion and memory loss.

Major Tranquilizers and Memory Loss

In the last chapter we discussed the effects of bromides, barbiturates, and tranquilizers in depressing memory function and decreasing memory abilities. The tranquilizers we discussed were the so-called minor tranquilizers, which are routinely given to people who have agitation or panic attacks.

The major tranquilizers, such as the phenothiazines — including Thorazine, Prolixin, Compazine, Mellaril, and Stelazine — produce much more severe brain dysfunction and memory loss than the minor tranquilizers. These agents (used mainly on profoundly agitated, hallucinating, delusional psychiatric patients) can cause symptoms very much like those of Parkinson's disease: an inability to initiate movement, a masklike facial expression, a shuffling gait, and slowness of movement.

A great number of people who take this kind of drug for a period of time develop a disorder of the central nervous system called tardive dyskinesia. This syndrome, which begins weeks to months after the agent is first administered, consists of involuntary movements of the face or tongue, with occasional tonic spasms of the legs and arms. These complications can occur after even an initial dose of the medication, although that's rare. More often the abnormal movements of the face, tongue, and neck occur late and become persistent complications. Occasionally these agents produce a catatonic rigidity and stupor.

Related drugs like haloperidol (Haldol) have much the same antipsychotic effects as the phenothiazines. They may also have the same kinds of side effects, and they do tend to cause severe interruptions of thought and memory which are oftentimes dose-dependent. Reducing or eliminating this drug will reduce its toxic effects on thinking and memory, but often a decrease in dosage will precipitate a recurrence of the original symptoms, including hallucinations, that first prompted the use of this agent. Of course, the movement disorders described as tardive dyskinesia may persist even after the drug has been completely discontinued.

Antidepressants and Memory Loss

Another class of psychoactive drugs, many of which have different chemical characteristics, are the antidepressants. It is not my purpose to discourage people from using psychoactive drugs if they are necessary in treating psychiatric disease. Severe depression is certainly an indication for their use. It is important to realize, however, that not all psychoactive drugs have the same effects or act through the same mechanisms. This is particularly true with antidepressants, as the following story illustrates.

Molly, a fifty-seven-year-old advertising copywriter who was subject to depression, was referred to me by her psychiatrist when she began to have symptoms of memory loss. She had difficulty performing her complex job because she couldn't keep all the variables and facets of her responsibility in focus. Because of her chronic depression she was taking a drug called Elavil, which had been very effective. More recently her doses of the agent had been slightly increased to give her the same therapeutic effect, and that's when she began to suffer memory loss.

Elavil not only improves the mood; it also has the effect of interfering with the acetylcholine network in the brain. Realizing that Molly needed to be on an antidepressant, I suggested that her psychiatrist change her to Prozac. Not all antidepressants are equally effective in treating the symptoms of a given patient, and there has to be a certain amount of trial and error to see whether the patient will respond to any one of them. Molly had responded to Elavil, and she also responded to Prozac — and this antidepressant was less toxic to Molly's memory function than Elavil.

You should not get the idea from this example that Elavil is not a useful drug and that Prozac is; the effectiveness of any drug depends on the unique biochemistry of each patient. The Prozac relieved Molly's depression and did not impair her memory, although there was no way of knowing what the result of her taking the drug would be before she tried it. (Incidentally, double-blind crossover experiments have shown that Elavil has a slightly greater tendency to impair intellectual and memory functions than does Prozac.) The point in my telling you this story is not to recommend one antidepressant over another, but merely to indicate that it is possible to substitute one medication for another when each has similar therapeutic effects on the user but is tolerated quite differently.

However, there is no perfect antidepressant, though some have fewer side effects than others. Elavil, for example, one of a class of drugs known as the tricyclic antidepressants, often causes people taking it to experience dryness in their mouths, constipation, dizziness (particularly when standing up quickly), weight gain, and sleepiness. Others may experience increased sensitivity to the sun, confusion, and even agitation. Prozac, even though it is generally thought to produce fewer side effects, can bring about nervousness, diarrhea, headaches, drowsiness, and insomnia, depending on the individual. Before you take either of these drugs — or any drug, for that matter — it's always wise to know as much about the possible long- and short-term side effects as you can.

The treatment of people who have been brain-poisoned by one medication is not simply to take them off all medications; doing so would also deprive them of needed therapy. Rather, the solution is to carefully titrate and adjust the dosage of the medication causing the problem, and if that doesn't work then to shift medications cautiously to try to find one that works without producing toxicity.

Monitoring Potentially Dangerous Situations

Certain combinations of drugs, like Mellaril and lithium or haloperidol and the antihypertensive drug methyldopa, are known to be particularly likely to produce memory loss and other forms of intellectual deterioration and even a confusional state. Also, a number of medicines that supposedly have nothing to do with the brain can cause rather pronounced alteration of mental function or loss of memory. This is why it's important to have a single knowledgeable physician to monitor all the medications you take — not just psychiatric or brain medications but also medications for the heart, lungs, kidneys, and so on. Your doctor must make sure that you are not becoming intoxicated or, in particular, brain-poisoned. This physician may have to contact your other specialists if a change in medications is necessary so that important drug therapies are not disturbed.

If you don't have a single physician monitoring your medications, it is possible that each of the specialists you see will write a prescription for a drug to treat one or another part of your body. You might end up with a heart medication, glaucoma medication, antihypertensive medication, and then possibly a sedative. All of these medications may affect your brain function and specifically your memory. Sometimes the combination of drugs is more poisonous to your brain than a single drug alone. Psychiatrists who specialize in psychopharmacology may be able to measure the toxic effects of all of the agents you take. But if a psychiatrist is your principal physician, he or she must be in communication with your other doctors and be aware of other prescription medications you take which are not associated with the brain but can impair brain function and memory.

Antihypertensive Drugs and Memory Loss

Just as with the antidepressant drugs, antihypertensive agents may have various effects on memory and intellectual capacity. Again, this phenomenon is individualized. Antihypertensive agents that are beta blockers, like Propranalol and Atenolol, may decrease memory performance more consis-

91

tently than antihypertensive agents that act through a different mechanism, such as angiotensin-converting enzyme inhibitors like Enalapril, which have very little effect on memory.

Some of the drugs that can impair memory include digitalis preparations, drugs to relieve pain, antihypertensive agents (as we've discussed), and any agent that depresses the level of blood glucose, especially those for treatment of diabetes. Eye drops for glaucoma, and even gastrointestinal drugs like cimetidine, may produce a loss of memory and interfere with other intellectual functions.*

Polypharmacy

It's always a challenge to go into a nursing home to review a patient who has had a recent decrease in memory abilities and intellectual function. Of course, after ruling out obvious physical problems that may affect the brain, I always try to find out whether the person has had a recent depression or change in mood. Next I look at the medications the patient is on. Often I am dismayed because many patients were started on several medications and, as time went by, one medication was added to another, with none of them ever stopped. This is what we call polypharmacy.

Jim, a retired mechanic who came to see me from Connecticut, was such a patient. He had a long list of the medications he took, and the doctors who prescribed these medicines weren't particularly concerned about their effects on the brain because none of the drugs were primarily for brain problems. And yet Jim had an obvious decrease in memory abilities and intellectual capacity from the combined effects of all these

*A relevant case here is that of President Bush, who was diagnosed in early 1990 as having a mild case of glaucoma in one eye for which eye drops were prescribed. Shortly after making the diagnosis, his doctors put him on the new medication but they quickly took him off it, possibly because they realized that the drops might adversely affect his judgment or memory.

medications. It was then a matter of trial and error in slowly decreasing the dosages of those drugs that might be inessential to see if we could uncover the guilty culprit or culprits — that is, the drug or combination of drugs that had such a toxic effect on Jim's brain function.

In Jim's case it turned out to be three different medications: one for his heart, one for his high blood pressure, and one for asthma. What my associates and I tried to do was cut out those medications that could be dispensed with and substitute others at lower dosages to treat the medical conditions that required continuous therapy. Obviously we were not so zealous in reducing his medication that he would develop any symptoms of undertreated disease.

Besides his supportive family, Jim had a cooperative and concerned physician who had initially referred him to our Center for Memory Impairment. His doctor began to carry out our recommendations — slowly, in order to avoid the toxic effects of abrupt withdrawal of medications. At the same time, he substituted medications that were less toxic to Jim than the ones he had been taking. After Jim's third trip to the Center for Memory Impairment, he was dramatically improved without suffering any side effects because appropriate medications had been substituted to treat his heart condition, his high blood pressure, and his asthma.

Antiemetics and Seasickness Medications

I'd like to say a word to all the sailors reading this who have a tendency to get seasick. Some people who are prone to motion sickness often use transdermal patches applied behind their ears which infuse a medication that masks the symptoms of *mal de mer*. If the medication is scopolamine, they'd better be cautious about sailing because this drug can have a negative effect on memory and other intellectual functions.

At one time, particularly in the late twenties, women in the throes of childbirth were often given large doses of scopolamine. This drug was prescribed because it didn't inhibit uterine contractions and at the same time was supposed to make them more comfortable. Actually it didn't do much for their comfort. But when they were questioned after the event, they had very few complaints about how their obstetrical management was handled. In fact, they had no memory of the event at all; the scopolamine had completely wiped out their memories. This phenomenon, then known as "twilight sleep," resulted from an interference with the acetylcholine mechanisms in the hippocampus which are essential in acquiring new memories.

Scopolamine has such a profound effect in reducing memory function that it is often used in a wide variety of medical experiments. But you should be aware that any agent used to reduce nausea or vertigo, and especially seasickness, may also have the tendency to adversely affect memory function. If you sail, you might not be able to make accurate nautical measurements and exercise superior seamanship and judgment if your memory circuits — those parts of the brain which are so necessary to any intellectual process — are working at half speed or less.

How and When to Talk to Your Doctor

The most important lesson you can draw from this chapter is that of the necessity of self-reliance. In the final analysis, it is you who consumes the prescription drugs, and it is you who must be responsible for preventing drug-induced impairment of your mind or memory. Your best safeguard against self-inflicted damage is to question your doctor carefully every time a new drug is prescribed or the dose is changed on one you are already taking. Your questions should include the following:

94

1. Why am I taking this drug?
2. Why do I need this drug?
3. Why is the dose being changed?
4. What are the toxic effects of this drug?
5. What are the effects of taking this drug for a long time?
6. Will this drug interfere with any other drug I'm taking?
7. Will this drug combine with another drug I'm taking to be more toxic than either alone?
8. Will this drug affect my mind or my memory?
9. How long will I be on this drug?
10. What toxic effects might arise if I discontinue taking this drug?

Remember, it is your life and brain function that are at stake. You deserve courteous and complete answers to your questions, and if you don't get them you may need another doctor.

Vital Memory Points to Remember

1. As we get older, our brain cells decrease in number and become more susceptible to brain poisoning.
2. There should be reduced dosage schedules of medications for people over age fifty-five.
3. Major tranquilizers can produce severe memory loss.
4. Some antidepressants may cause memory loss.
5. A single physician should be in charge of monitoring all your prescriptions in order to reduce the possibility of adverse side effects from their combination.

Diet and Reversible Memory Loss

YOUR BRAIN is a very sensitive organ requiring precise amounts of sugar, oxygen, water, sodium, potassium, and vitamins in order to function properly. If there isn't enough sugar or oxygen, or too much water, or insufficient nutrition (such as a lack of certain key vitamins), your brain function and especially your memory can deteriorate dramatically.

Many possible reasons can account for imbalances in our brains' support systems as we grow older. For example, with advancing age we are often less active. We therefore eat smaller amounts of food since we need fewer calories. That's not bad if with the decreased amount of food we receive sufficient vitamins, especially B vitamins. But for those of us who don't supplement our diets with vitamin pills this may not be the case. Good diets of 1,800 to 2,200 calories a day may not contain enough essential thiamine (vitamin B-1), for example, to replenish body stores, and vitamin B deficiencies may occur, particularly in times of stress.

Another reason we may not get enough B vitamins as we grow older is that we may lose teeth and not be able to chew food properly for thorough digestion of nutrients. And of course, if we have poor teeth, we are going to avoid foods we have to chew and take foods that are semisolid and go down easily. These foods may not contain enough B vitamins or even proteins.

In Chapter 9 I discuss only briefly what happens when all the nutrients obtained from the diet are reduced to dangerously low levels. Fortunately, such malnutrition is rare in the United States except in certain pockets of extreme poverty. The majority of the chapter describes the more likely scenario, namely an inadequate intake of some of the important B vitamins.

Chapter 10 describes some aspects of brain chemistry, focusing on concentrations of certain electrolytes and water which affect memory. The balancing of these substances is especially significant to us as we grow older since if we don't take in proper amounts of water and electrolytes during hot and humid days our brain function can be impaired.

Chapter 11 focuses on problems of memory that stem from a relative lack of oxygen and sugar in the arterial blood stream, and in turn in the capillary blood bringing oxygen and sugar to the brain cells.

So many mechanisms and controls have to work perfectly in order to keep intelligence and memory performing at optimal levels that it often seems a wonder our brains work as well as they do. To regulate these complicated processes, the human body has a series of checks and balances which in a delicate, sophisticated, and accurate way feed information back to control centers. These centers are part of the early warning, fail-safe mechanisms that usually prevent abnormalities from occurring and ensure that the brain, the most important organ in our bodies, is given top priority, along with the heart and lungs, in any stressful situation. Disease, injury, and chronic neglect can break down these fail-safe mechanisms, however, and cause intellectual and memory functions to decline. Understanding how some of these important mechanisms work will help us avoid potentially dangerous pitfalls.

9

Memory Loss Related to
Brain Nutrition

Is YOUR DIET adequate, or do you eat junk foods that are high in fat and loaded with salt? Can you chew your food properly, or are your teeth in such poor condition (or your plates so loose) that you give up on foods that need to be chewed thoroughly before they can be swallowed? Are you a food faddist, adopting the latest diet to lose weight and then rapidly gaining it all back, only to go on another crazy diet again, perhaps one requiring liquid protein supplements? Do you find that your appetite is fading and that you are eating less and less food?

If you fall into any of these categories you may have a nutritional deficiency that can affect your memory. A number of nutritional deficiency problems can alter vital memory, even in those of us who are generally not malnourished or protein-starved. For example, a deficiency in minerals like calcium, phosphorus, iodine, iron, magnesium, copper, or zinc can undermine mental functions. Also, the water-electrolyte balance must be kept in proper alignment. And, of course, vitamins — those substances our bodies do not produce but which are nevertheless essential to normal brain function — must be present in adequate amounts. Usually the amount of vitamins necessary to produce the desired beneficial effects is relatively small.

Vitamins A, D, E, C, and all the B vitamins (including biotin) play important roles in maintaining our brain processes. It is certain of the B vitamins which, when lacking or deficient in our diets, can most easily produce a loss of vital memory. I focus on three of them here: vitamin B-1, or thiamine; B-3, niacin or nicotinic acid; and B-12. Each of these three can have a most profound effect on our vital memory functions, and in fact on many other functions of our central nervous systems.

Choline is another compound that some investigators include among vitamins essential for memory. Choline is not technically a vitamin since it is partially synthesized in the body and is present in larger quantities than any of the true vitamins. It is a component of the acetylcholine molecule, the neurotransmitter that is a vital part of the memory circuits. Patients with Alzheimer's disease who have severe recent-memory loss tend to have reduced levels of acetylcholine in the inner part of their temporal lobes.

Researchers have tested the effects of increased choline intake in preventing symptoms of memory loss, both in those of us who are aging normally and also in Alzheimer's patients. Some studies have shown that large amounts of choline are helpful in certain kinds of memory function, but the evidence that increasing the amount of choline has any significant effect in improving the loss of recent memory in patients who do have Alzheimer's disease is less convincing.

If you want to try taking increased amounts of choline (something I do myself), I suggest you take it in a highly purified form called PhosChol, a brand name for concentrated lecithin. In my own case I've found it to be very helpful, and I believe that it produces a real improvement in memory rather than a placebo effect.

100

Food Sources of B Vitamins

How did primitive man survive and keep from being vitamin deficient when there were no supplemental vitamins around? The primary source of vitamin B-12 for ancient peoples was meat and other animal products. Through the action of bacteria, vitamin B-12 is present in beef, beef liver, eggs, flounder, herring, liverwurst, mackerel, milk, and milk products. With an adequate amount of animal products, including fish, in their diets, people won't develop vitamin B-12 deficiency unless their bodies lack what is known as the "intrinsic factor," a chemical discovered by two doctors at the Boston City Hospital which is present in gastric juice and whose role is to allow vitamin B-12 to be absorbed into the blood stream. If there is a lack or deficiency of this intrinsic factor, vitamin B-12 won't get into the blood stream even if the vitamin is plentiful in the food that's digested.

Conversely, even when an adequate amount of the intrinsic factor is available, vitamin B-12 deficiency will occur if there is not enough of the vitamin in the diet. This is the case with strict vegetarians because vitamin B-12 does not occur in vegetables or fruits, unless they are mixed with bacterial products in some way.

Niacin (vitamin B-3) too is present in many meat products: beef liver, the white meat of chicken, halibut, peanuts, pork, salmon, swordfish, tuna, turkey, and veal, as well as in brewer's yeast and sunflower seeds. Thiamine (vitamin B-1) occurs in beef kidney, beef liver, and especially in brewer's yeast, in addition to whole wheat flour, wheat germ, whole grain products, dried navy beans, rice bran, raw brown rice, salmon steak, and soybeans.

The requirements for certain B vitamins, especially thiamine, are increased with greater caloric intake, and that is especially true of the greater caloric intake associated with drinking large amounts of alcohol or alcohol products. Pellagra, a disease occurring when niacin is deficient, is more common in countries that depend on maize or corn as a principal element in the diet.

People who don't have a deficiency of the intrinsic factor in their gastrointestinal mucosa, and whose diets are normal, including the substances we have enumerated, are unlikely to have a deficiency in these three B vitamins. However, persons on a reducing diet, or elderly people whose dietary intake is compromised by poor teeth or lack of appetite, may require supplementation.*

The Major B Vitamins: Deficiency Syndromes Producing Memory Loss

Vitamin B-1 (Thiamine) Deficiency

Neurologists see many patients who are both alcohol abusers and victims of malnutrition. A number of them have persistent memory loss, even after they get massive vitamin therapy. Some neurologists got the idea that it might be possible to prevent some of the bad results of alcohol abuse by persuading the liquor, beer, and wine industries to add certain B vitamins to their beverages, and I went so far as to write a formal letter to one of the biggest distillers of alcohol, imploring the company to add thiamine to its product — an action that, if it were undertaken on a large scale, would save the

---

*Dietary supplements can be bought in any drug or food store. Mindful of the fact that elderly people who suffer no specific clinical syndrome are reluctant to see a physician about vitamin supplements and too often buy preparations that have excessive amounts of vitamins, Dr. Tom Sabin and I have devised our own vitamin preparation. The Schiff Company brought out the Neural Nutrient Formula in 1990 on our recommendation. The formula provides enough vitamins to avoid any deficiencies, even in times of stress, without overloading the system with foolishly excessive and unnecessary amounts of vitamins, which can have a detrimental effect. Additional lecithin is found in PhosChol, made by Advanced Nutritional Technology, 1111 Jefferson Avenue, Elizabeth, New Jersey 07207.

useful lives of many thousands of people every year. Unhap-pily, the company's directors didn't think this was necessary.*

Today, alcohol producers go right on making their potent brain poisons, which are consumed by millions of Americans on a regular basis, without any thought as to how they can reduce the damage. In a way they're almost worse than ciga-rette manufacturers, who at least put filters on their cigarettes to try to reduce the amount of tar and nicotine which is inhaled. But the liquor distilleries refuse to put thiamine in their products, or even package it separately and dispense it along with the beverages, which would help stop the mem-ory loss associated with this deficiency.

Helene was a victim of the liquor industry who was caught in time. A sixty-two-year-old retired secretary living in a mod-ern suburb with a small garden apartment and a failing mar-riage, she had blunted her emotional disappointment with an increasing daily ration of white wine, and subsequently vodka (vodka because she was under the impression that it did not leave a detectable odor on her breath). She would begin drinking early in the morning and often neglected to eat. On several occasions her husband had committed her to a mental hospital for the treatment of alcohol abuse, but when she came home she would start drinking and starving herself, just as she had before.

One morning Helene's cleaning lady found her confused and irrational, called the police ambulance, and had her taken to the local hospital. It was several days before the doctors there called in a neurologist. He found her to be confused and apathetic, and she was suffering from nystagmus, an unusual jiggling of the eyeballs when she tried to look from one side to the other. The neurologist also found that Helene

*Federal regulations against adding vitamins directly to brain poisons such as alcoholic beverages could be overcome by attaching packages of B vitamin capsules to each bottle of alcoholic beverage.

had lost a substantial amount of recent memory. After his examination he sent her to one of the large hospitals, where I saw her.

I found Helene's loss of recent memory to be extensive and very disabling. What tipped me off to the true nature of her confusional state, however, was some of the answers she gave to my questions. At first I discounted them because I thought they simply reflected her confusion. But then it became obvious that her statements had fictional elements that confusion alone couldn't explain.

She told me, for example, that she had six children, although her husband had previously informed me that the couple was childless. She told me that she and her husband lived in a grand mansion in one of the most fashionable suburbs of Chicago, Illinois, but I found that her garden apartment in a suburb of Boston was modest, and that she and her husband barely scraped by because of some of the reckless and unpredictable expenditures she incurred under the influence of alcohol.

These tall tales constitute a clinical symptom called confabulation, and together with her abnormal eye movement and the profound loss of recent memory, the diagnosis of Wernicke's Korsakoff's psychosis and thiamine deficiency was a certainty. This diagnosis was based on the history of inadequate food and vitamin intake that often occurs in patients who consume an excessive amount of alcohol. The clinical syndrome involving abnormal eye movement and the subsequent loss of recent memory are typical of Wernicke's disease. Unfortunately, most victims of this disease have suffered significant and irreversible damage to the inner parts of their thalamus and hypothalamus.

Two neurologists working at the Boston City Hospital and the Massachusetts General, Maurice Victor and Ray Adams, spent years examining patients with vitamin deficiency and alcoholism. They and other researchers indicated that the principal culprit resulting in the destruction of the patients' vital memories, particularly their recent-memory functions, was a lack of thiamine. The patients simply couldn't remember one fact or incident that exceeded their attention span. When the attention shifted, recent memory disappeared.

Although it is rare, some patients had a combined deficiency of vitamins B-5 (pantothenic acid) and B-6 (pyridoxine) as well as a thiamine deficiency. I suspected that this might have been the case with Helene, so I treated her with massive doses of all three B vitamins, both intravenously and by mouth. After a short while she was able to take other nutritious foods as well. The clinical result was favorable in Helene's case because there was a rapid resolution of most of her signs and symptoms, including a return of her vital memory, with only a modest loss of recent memory.

It was lucky for Helene that she was treated promptly. Most patients with persistent symptoms such as hers do not get their memory functions back, even when they're given an adequate course of treatment with the B vitamins, because lasting structural damage has taken place in the center of their brains which makes memory loss permanent. That's why it's so important to get the message across to wineries, beer manufacturers, and especially distilleries: if you're going to sell brain poisons like alcohol, at least put some B vitamins in them or attach them to the bottle to reduce the bad effects. Adding vitamins wouldn't prevent cirrhosis of the liver or its associated bleeding from the esophagus, but at least it would slow down brain deterioration.

Finally, I want to emphasize again that thiamine deficiency is in itself more important than alcohol abuse in causing memory loss. Severe thiamine deficiency, without alcohol abuse, has at times caused memory loss, although in our society such cases are unusual, and thiamine deficiency alone generally produces peripheral neuritis and numbness as its most outstanding features.

Pellagra: Vitamin B-3 (Niacin) Deficiency

At one time state mental hospitals were inhabited by a lot of patients who were all classified as "crazy." The leading cause of their insanity was not schizophrenia or manic-depression; it was syphilis of the brain, an infectious disorder transmitted by a spirochete that produces a serious loss of many brain functions. The second leading cause was not an infection but a deficiency disease called pellagra, which tends to affect persons eating a diet consisting mostly of corn or maize since these foods do not supply enough niacin to meet the body's needs.

Today pellagra is unusual in the United States because many of the foods we buy in the supermarket, particularly most commercially baked breads, have added niacin. Pellagra is now largely restricted to underdeveloped countries, especially among the black population of South Africa.

I still remember my father, a general practitioner, showing me one of his patients, a farmer whom he treated in his practice back in the Great Depression. I was particularly struck by the man's lesions on areas of his skin exposed to sunlight.

This sick farmer had a couple of other important symptoms. He complained of abdominal cramps and diarrhea, and his wife said that he was depressed and didn't respond very well, and he kept forgetting what he had to do around the farm. One other thing worried her most of all. She turned to my father and said, "Do you think he's going mental?"

My father didn't then know that pellagra was a disease caused by a deficiency of niacin; when he saw this man, niacin hadn't yet been identified. He did know, however, that it was a deficiency disease, and he put the farmer on milk, yeast, and liver — foods he paid for out of his own pocket. The man's mental symptoms quickly disappeared.

Now, of course, we know that this disorder can be treated

with niacin. Sometimes pyridoxine (vitamin B-6) is also needed to reverse the symptoms completely.

Vitamin B-12 Deficiency

A deficiency of vitamin B-12 can occur in the body even though an individual has an adequate diet. A special factor present in the gastric juice, the intrinsic factor, allows vitamin B-12 in our food to be absorbed into the blood stream. When this factor is missing, we can have a vitamin B-12 deficiency even though there's plenty of this vitamin in our food.

When vitamin B-12, along with folic acid, is deficient, a disease called pernicious anemia results. This condition is associated with combined degeneration of the spinal cord as well as a disease of the brain. The anemia can be cured with folic acid, but only vitamin B-12 can cure the diseases affecting the brain and spinal cord, which can produce numbness, spasticity and weakness of the muscles, signs of brain changes ranging from irritability to apathy and emotional instability, and finally a great loss of vital memory, with confusion or intellectual deterioration.

There are methods of measuring levels of vitamin B-12 in the blood. Classical nutritionists determined standards of what sufficient amounts of this vitamin were, without which an individual might get spinal cord disease or severe brain disease, including dementia and memory loss. Recent studies have shown, however, that the classical nutritionists set their standards too low, and that even when the amount of vitamin B-12 in the blood falls in the low-normal range, major neurobehavioral symptoms, including apathy, can occur.

Hildy was a twenty-three-year-old graduate student who was almost fanatical about avoiding any kind of poison — cigarettes, alcohol, or any sort of tainted food — and was also a strict vegetarian. She began to have symptoms of fatigue and memory loss, which were troublesome to her in her quite demanding studies. Eventually she came to see me, complaining of serious recent memory loss.

A complete evaluation disclosed that her vitamin B-12 level was in the low-normal range. She was not lacking the so-called intrinsic factor, which promotes the absorption of vitamin B-12 into her blood stream; rather, Hildy was one of those vegetarians who just don't get enough vitamin B-12 in their diets. I wasn't surprised at this because vegetarians, unless their food is contaminated by bacteria, have little if any of this vitamin in their diets. In Hildy's case, her vitamin B-12 level wasn't high enough to allow her brain to function normally. The addition of supplemental vitamin B-12 to her diet was enough to reverse her symptoms, disperse her depression, and improve her memory.

I'd like to stress this point to all vegetarians: if you're faithful to a regime of no meat or fish, you'll get very little if any vitamin B-12. This is an essential vitamin, and you must take vitamin supplements to maintain your nutritional balance. You may not feel in any way deficient or ill now, but once your body's store of vitamin B-12 is used up you'll run into precisely the same problems Hildy did. Moreover, people with pale blue eyes and a lack of hydrochloric acid in their stomachs are more likely than others to get pernicious anemia, a tendency that may be genetically determined. Such patients lack the intrinsic factor, and for them vitamin B-12 must be given by intramuscular injection — oral supplements are not effective.

A Balanced Diet and Vitamin Supplements

I'm often asked whether it's a good idea for those of us who eat a so-called balanced diet to take vitamin supplements, particularly of the B vitamins. In my opinion, because many of us eat less food as we grow older since we are less active and burn fewer calories, it is wise to add essential vitamins to make up for our reduced intake from the foods we eat.

I don't recommend megavitamin consumption because most of the excess vitamins are excreted in the urine and toxic concentrations of others can result. But based on what I've seen in my own medical practice, I believe that most people can benefit from taking larger amounts of vitamins — larger, that is, than the amounts recommended by classical nutritionists. I discuss in detail what I think are optimal levels of vitamins for various age groups in a subsequent chapter.

Finally, chemical tests of your blood can be carried out to determine whether or not you have an adequate concentration of B vitamins in your blood stream. Unless you have symptoms of Korsakoff's psychosis or beriberi, vitamin B-12 and folate are the vitamins usually tested for. These tests can be carried out by your doctor, and you may also consult with either your physician or a nutritionist to determine the proper dose of vitamin supplements you need. Most vitamin supplements contain extra vitamins that you may or may not need. There is a real danger of taking too much of certain vitamins, particularly the fat-soluble ones, which may have negative effects on your health. A doctor or nutritionist can help you avoid these complications. In addition, your doctor may prescribe extra vitamins if you are on any medicine that can deplete vitamin reserves, such as Dilantin, which uses up the body's store of vitamin D and, at times, certain B vitamins.

The routine laboratory tests we carry out on every patient who complains of memory loss include a hemogram with red blood cell indices to identify, for example, pernicious anemia, with associated folate and vitamin B-12 deficiencies. Most physicians conduct these examinations twice a year on their elderly patients, so a diagnosis of pernicious anemia is not likely to be missed. The isolated deficiency of vitamin B-12, however, is more likely to be undiagnosed, which is why we prescribe vitamin B-12 injections for our memory loss patients, even when their vitamin B-12 levels are in the low-normal range.

Vital Memory Points to Remember

1. As you get older and require fewer calories, you may need extra vitamins to replenish body stores.
2. Many elderly people don't get enough B vitamins.
3. A lack of vitamin B-1, B-3, or B-12 can readily produce a loss of vital memory.
4. Strict vegetarians *must* take supplements of vitamin B-12.

10

The Chemistry of the Body and How It Affects the Mind (Especially Vital Memory)

Electrolytes and the Brain

IF YOU'VE EVER BEEN with a very elderly or sick person when he or she became dehydrated, especially on a hot and humid day when fluid and electrolytes are lost through the lungs and skin and aren't replaced, you've noticed that the person began to have changes in mental functioning. One of the first problems encountered is a loss of memory. This happened to Muriel, one of my patients. Fortunately, I was there to observe the changes and reverse them with proper treatment.

Muriel, seventy-eight, a retired office administrator, was a slender, white-haired lady who was in the hospital to be treated with antibiotics for lung infection that interfered with her breathing. Massive doses of antibiotics had conquered the infection and she seemed to be on the road to recovery, but I was asked to examine her neurologically because one of her doctors thought she had a mental problem.

When I first saw her, about nine o'clock one morning, I carried out the routine tests, which showed her mental status functions — particularly her memory — to be normal. But because of the press of my schedule that day, I couldn't finish my examination, and I told her I'd be back after noon.

111

Muriel was in a two-bed hospital room without air conditioning. Mid-July in Boston can be hot, humid, and extremely uncomfortable. When I returned to examine her around 2:00 P.M., five hours later, I found that she had undergone a profound change in mental function, and her recent memory had declined to zero out of three.

At first I couldn't understand what might have produced this dramatic change in Muriel's mental abilities. Was her pneumonia worse, was she coughing, was she feverish, did she have trouble breathing? None of these was the answer.

What had happened was that Muriel was scheduled to have a special chest x ray, and through some miscommunication the nursing staff thought she was to have nothing by mouth before the exam. Over a five-hour period of intense heat and humidity in the hospital room, Muriel received no fluids; in fact, she hadn't eaten or drunk anything since nine o'clock the previous evening. A check of her blood electrolytes showed that her body water was depleted and that the concentration of sodium in her serum was extremely elevated.

Dehydration can actually produce shrinkage of the brain, and besides the kind of mental changes I found in Muriel, the patient may become very irritable. If she hadn't been treated promptly, she might have had even worse problems, including stupor. Because she was somewhat nauseated it was thought best to replace her deficient fluids intravenously. An IV infusion was done slowly because too rapid a correction of fluid imbalance can cause problems in other organ systems, and even in the brain itself.

The slow replacement of Muriel's fluids and electrolytes, giving her small amounts of potassium in a very dilute solution, brought her blood chemistry back to normal. Her depleted potassium rose, and her excessive sodium concentration slowly decreased to the normal range. Her nausea disappeared, and she was able to supplement the intravenous fluids by drinking appropriately buffered, not too distasteful liquid concoctions. Two days later she returned to her usual state of health and brain function and was discharged.

Most of us have had the experience of mental fatigue and slight memory problems, or even of feeling faint, while working or exercising in hot and humid weather. We have also been told on radio and television to drink extra fluids in such conditions and consume salt pills or drinks like Gatorade which contain potassium. If we don't replace fluids and electrolytes in a timely fashion, it should not surprise us that our symptoms will be severe.

In fact, confusion and even stupor may result when the concentration of various ions, or electrolytes, in the serum of the blood that irrigates the brain becomes unbalanced. When that imbalance affects the fluids surrounding the brain cells, and particularly the membranes of those brain cells, the most severe reactions occur, as happened to Muriel.

Although some neurologists find no evidence that memory itself is compromised in confusional states, when orientation to time, place, and even person is lacking, I contend that this state represents a severe loss of vital memory. The fact that the clinical syndromes associated with electrolyte imbalance may progress to stupor or even coma, on the one hand, or hyperirritability and epileptic seizures, on the other, indicates the importance of electrolyte concentrations, particularly across the membranes of nerve cells and brain fibers.

What Electrolytes and Ions Do

An electrolyte is a chemical that in a solution such as water, or especially blood, dissociates into ions. These ions have a small electric charge, either positive or negative, and are found both inside and outside the membranes of nerve cells and fibers. They help control the excitability of nerve elements and the conduction and propagation of electrical impulses in nerve fibers. The actual concentration of ions

113

within and around nerve cells depends to some extent on the concentration of ions in the serum of the blood that circulates to and from the brain.

There are a number of important ions, such as sodium, potassium, chloride, calcium, magnesium, and carbonate, whose concentration can fluctuate only within a small range if the brain cells and brain mechanisms are to function properly. In a normal person, eating a nutritious diet and drinking sufficient but not excessive amounts of fluid ensure that the homeostatic regulation of ions and electrolytes is within normal limits. The acid-base balance is regulated in the same way, as described later in this chapter.

Probably the most important ion in the human body is the sodium ion. Its concentration in both the blood and the brain is related to the amount of water in and around the cells, particularly brain cells. When water becomes less plentiful, the concentration of sodium ion can increase dramatically, which may result in serious memory loss and rapid decline in mental abilities.

The reverse problem of too much water in the body can also occur, especially in hot weather when people perspire freely, losing salt in their perspiration and replacing it only with water or, as sometimes happens at sporting events, large amounts of beer. This overhydration can produce swelling of tissues and even of the brain. Again, not only vital memory but other aspects of mental function can be deranged. Drowsiness, giddiness, headaches, and nausea are quite common. Some people, especially those who are seizure-prone, may suffer convulsions if they become too waterlogged without taking in sufficient amounts of salt.

How do you tell whether major changes in electrolyte levels, and a loss of brain function possibly resulting in confusion, have occurred in elderly people, who may already be somewhat confused? They may have had memory loss or other symptoms that put them into the hospital or nursing home in the first place. The most important feature of diagnosis is a good history. In other words, establishing a neurological base line of the patient's function is critical so that one can determine if there is a change in personality, a worsening of intellectual abilities, or an increase in memory loss. If these things occur definitely and rather quickly, as happened with Muriel, a previous recent neurological evaluation will point that out. In her case, I was able to act quickly and decisively because I was certain that her neurological status indicated a change for the worse, and blood tests confirmed that she had an electrolyte and water imbalance.

Low Sodium Syndrome

One other note on low serum sodium syndrome, which is just the reverse of Muriel's problem. This syndrome can occur in severely head-injured patients because of inappropriate hormonal secretion, particularly of the antidiuretic hormone from the posterior pituitary. Patients who have this problem excrete urine that is supersaturated with sodium, but they retain water and quickly develop low sodium levels in their blood and around their nerve cell membranes. This condition exacerbates their brain problems and makes them susceptible to confusion, coma, and epileptic seizures.

You mainly need to concern yourself with electrolyte levels if:

- you are elderly and subjected to long spells of hot weather
- you are on a special diet — for example, a low-salt diet — and live in an excessively warm environment
- you are taking medicines that may cause a change in your electrolyte levels (ask your doctor about this)
- you are chronically ill and are subjected to stressful circumstances

115

If you fall in one of these four categories, consult your doctor. Let your doctor treat you — don't try to treat yourself. Ask for advice on the amount and kind of fluids which are right for you. If your doctor is in doubt, a simple blood test will determine whether or not you have an electrolyte imbalance. Your doctor can correct the imbalance by administering fluids or the electrolytes you are deficient in.

The Acid-Base Balance

The acid-base balance in and around the brain depends to some extent on the relationship between carbon dioxide and bicarbonate concentrations in the blood. Changes in the acid-base balance, for example in disease states such as diabetic coma, in which an increase in acidity occurs, affect brain function and memory. Acid-base imbalance is only one form of metabolic imbalance. A number of diverse disorders can produce such imbalances, and these disorders, which secondarily derange brain function, have their origin in the malfunction of other organ systems in the body, including the heart, lungs, kidney, liver, pancreas, and endocrine glands.

The acid-base imbalance is a relatively common metabolic disturbance that frequently causes brain dysfunction, or at least temporary deterioration in brain function, and loss of memory.

This imbalance is commonly experienced by people when they overbreathe when they're not actually working or running or exercising, and they blow off too much carbon dioxide as well as reduce the ionized calcium in their serum. They feel giddy and extremely dizzy. If one tests their mental status during this time there is a decrease in certain mental functions, including memory, as is illustrated in the case of Carrie, a thirty-seven-year-old mother of four.

One Saturday morning as she was pushing her shopping cart through the aisles of a supermarket, Carrie noticed that she was getting dizzy. If she hadn't had the shopping cart to

116

lean on she would have fallen down. Moreover, she didn't know what items to select from the shelf. (She had never had this trouble before; her memory was good enough that she never used a shopping list.)

As Carrie became increasingly dizzy and confused she got a tingling sensation in her fingers, and she panicked. She ran out of the store and sat in her car for a long while until she gradually recovered. She was obviously disturbed by the mysterious ailment, but she didn't seek medical help until it happened again a short time after that. When it happened a third time she was referred to me to rule out some seizure disorder.

Carrie did not have seizures, and all her brain tests were normal. What she did have was a disturbance in her acid-base balance because she was hyperventilating and blowing off a large amount of carbon dioxide. The reason she was hyperventilating was that, because of problems with her husband, she was suddenly under a great deal of stress and in a state of emotional turmoil.

If you want to know how Carrie felt, all you have to do is breathe in and out rapidly and deeply for one to three minutes, and you'll begin to notice the same dizziness and fuzziness. Actually it's not necessary to overbreathe purposely to achieve this result. If you have a feeling of being trapped, you may begin to overbreathe quite unconsciously but with the same result.

The treatment of Carrie's acid-base problem was quite simple. All she had to do was to hold her breath. And if she couldn't do that she could hold a paper bag over her mouth so that she could rebreathe her own carbon dioxide. Dealing with the stress that made her overbreathe in the first place was the next thing she had to work on.

If you ever have an acid-base problem from overbreathing, you can quickly reverse the dizziness and fuzzy mental function by heeding the advice I gave to Carrie. Just stop breathing for a short while, or hold a paper bag over your mouth until the symptoms disappear.

Homeostasis and Memory

Although homeostatic mechanisms exist in the brain, and although the pituitary and other endocrine glands secrete hormones to keep the water and electrolyte balance within a very narrow range of normal, dietary excess and dietary deficiency can change these concentrations, producing a decrease in many mental functions, including memory. Foods therefore must contain a sufficient amount of sodium, potassium, chloride, calcium, and magnesium, and intake of water should be adequate.

Normal concentration of water and electrolytes depends on proper excretion as well as adequate intake. In other words, a dysfunction or malfunction in the kidneys can cause a retention of waste products such as urea in the blood as well as an elevation of potassium. Routine chemical tests of your blood can determine whether you have this condition. If you have memory problems, make sure your doctor does these tests. Unfortunately for Laurence, his doctor did not do them in time.

Laurence was an eighty-two-year-old insurance salesman who had a probable case of Parkinson's disease, advancing rather slowly over a five- to six-year period. He was living in his own apartment with some occasional nursing assistance. Although he had problems orienting himself when he walked around the block, he was able to converse over the telephone and even talk knowledgeably about the stock exchange (and, incidentally, predict more accurately what was going to happen to the Dow Jones industrial average than some of the financial pundits seen on national television).

Laurence also had an enlarging prostate, which kept him from emptying his bladder. Over a period of time, urinary retention caused a dilatation of his ureters and finally a backup of urine into the kidneys themselves, which began to fail. Laurence didn't complain about his symptoms, and his doctor didn't pick up on his condition until he became comatose, his serum potassium level greatly elevated. He was rushed to the hospital, his bladder was emptied, and finally he had a prostate operation to relieve the obstruction. He did recover, but his mental function never returned to its previous level.

The brain of a person with Parkinson's disease is more fragile than that of a normal individual of the same age. It is a brain that withstands insult much less well than a normal brain. Laurence's doctor's failure to notice a medical problem superimposed on brain disease is not uncommon, but it reveals an attitude that must be changed in the medical profession.

Finally, Laurence's kidney deterioration might not have progressed as far and still produced an increased level of circulating potassium which would affect brain function adversely. Even an increase in the blood urea nitrogen may be associated with a decrease in memory function and some deterioration in intellectual ability. That's why it's critical to make certain that the dangers of urinary obstruction are appreciated and that medical or surgical means are used to correct it promptly.

The Importance of Homeostasis

To recap, the state of equilibrium called homeostasis results from feedback from regulatory processes in the brain, pituitary, and other organs such as the kidneys. These processes control the concentration of sodium, potassium, chloride, calcium, carbonate, and phosphate in the blood and in and around brain cells within very narrow limits. They also regulate the amount of water in and around brain cells as well as in other parts of the body.

Homeostasis of water and electrolytes in and around brain

cells is essential because any deviation above or below the normal concentrations may result in altered brain function, even in people who are otherwise normal. That this effect is more pronounced in cases of brain disease or injury is not only because the diseased brain is more susceptible to damage, but also because those homeostatic mechanisms originating in the brain may be deficient or absent. Maintaining water and electrolyte balance by adequate fluid and electrolyte administration in the elderly, particularly if they have symptoms of brain dysfunction, is essential.

The point I want to stress here is that homeostatic mechanisms may be more fragile in your elderly parent or relative, and they are more easily disrupted by disease states, particularly those affecting the brain. If the homeostatic mechanisms are fragile, your loved one must make a special effort to compensate. A person can do so by judicious intake of water and electrolytes, which is particularly important at times of stress — on very hot days, for example.

Even in completely healthy individuals like you and me, the body's homeostatic mechanisms can break down under conditions of extreme stress: when running a marathon, say, or crossing the Sahara, or climbing a peak in the Himalayas. Otherwise the mechanisms work well most of the time for people in good physical condition. The body is generally completely self-regulating, continually sending messages to the brain when it needs food, water, or oxygen. Homeostasis keeps the body chemistry at optimal levels of functioning all the time, until some extreme force or forces upset the balance. When that happens, it's usually wisest to seek immediate medical assistance.

If you faint on a hot day, or begin looking gray, or feel clammy and sick, ask your doctor to see you as an emergency patient in the office, or have your physician meet you at the emergency room of your local hospital. If you can't locate your doctor, the emergency room physician on duty is your best bet. If you or someone you know has collapsed, call an ambulance. The police or fire department will need to get you to the hospital for immediate treatment.

Vital Memory Points to Remember

1. An electrolyte is a chemical that, in solution, dissociates into ions. Sodium, potassium, chloride, calcium, magnesium, and carbonate are some of the important ions.
2. When someone in fragile health takes too much or too little water, a temporary electrolyte imbalance can occur which can cause memory loss.
3. The acid-base balance in the blood depends on carbon dioxide and bicarbonate concentrations.
4. Hyperventilation is the most common way that acid-base balance is disturbed.

11

Memory and Brain Metabolism

HAVE YOU EVER SEEN a very sick friend or relative with severe heart, lung, or liver disease — severe enough that the person had failing memory and intellect or delirium and stupor? And were you told that this deterioration was happening even though there was nothing intrinsically wrong with the person's brain? Such cases occur, not infrequently, illustrating that the brain does not work independently. Many organs of the body, especially the heart, which pumps blood to the brain, and other organs such as the liver, kidneys, lungs, and endocrine glands, must function adequately in order to support the activities of the brain. If you have a disorder of one of these organ systems and suffer failing memory or a loss of intellectual abilities, consult your physician for diagnosis and treatment because symptoms in this case often reflect a medical problem. Taking corrective actions on your own is apt to be counterproductive.

Blood Sugar and Vital Memory
Central to normal brain function are the life-giving nutrients: sugar, ketone bodies, and the oxygen necessary to metabolize them. Blood sugar levels are sensitive to ingested simple sugars so that it is possible, by eating large amounts

of simple sugars, to drive blood sugar up to very high levels, producing an insulin response. For the most part, however, blood sugar level is the result of complex metabolic mechanisms.

Sugar in the blood results from the breakdown of a number of complex foods containing, among other things, large carbohydrate molecules such as starch as well as amino acids. The degradation of amino acid carbon skeletons occurs in the liver, which converts these skeletons to glucose. By a different metabolic route the carbon skeletons can be converted to fatty acids, or to what are known as ketone bodies. Glucose and ketone bodies can be directly metabolized in the brain, although ketone bodies are also metabolized by muscles.

The brain's major fuel in a nonstarving human being on a mixed diet is glucose. In starvation states, ketone bodies are also used as fuel by the brain.

You don't need to understand the complexities of how sugars are metabolized, or what the body uses for fuel, but you should know that the concentration of sugar in the blood is normally kept within certain finite limits. If it's too high, as in diabetes mellitus, where insulin is insufficient, sugar and ketone bodies are spilled into the urine and the acid-base balance in the blood is disturbed. Severe acidosis then occurs which, if it persists, will result in diabetic coma.

Of course, vital memory is destroyed by any condition that can cause coma. The treatment for diabetes involves both an adequate amount of sugar and the right dosage of insulin. Since the treatment of patients in diabetic coma is usually handled by an internist and not a surgeon, I wasn't thinking about the treatment of diabetic coma when I went to sleep one night in the interns' quarters at the University of Minnesota Hospital.

I had been on duty for thirty-six continuous hours, most of which I spent in the operating room. The intern who had the bed next to mine (his last name also began with an *M*) was on the internal medicine rotation, in the service specializing in treating patients with diabetic coma.

I had only been asleep for fifteen or twenty minutes when the telephone rang, and my first thought as I answered the phone was that some emergency must have come up in one of my surgical cases. The head nurse I talked with said that the patient (I couldn't get the name) was in a diabetic coma, and I proceeded to give her instructions about the amounts of insulin and glucose needed to treat the patient. She called me about every thirty to thirty-five minutes during the rest of the night. As soon as I finished each conversation with her I would go back to sleep, only to have the telephone awaken me with another request for instructions.

I was more than a little baffled the next morning when my medical neighbor, the doctor whose last name also began with the letter *M*, thanked me profusely. "Gee," he said, "you did a beautiful job of treating my patient with diabetic coma. She's alert and bright as a penny now." I was astonished, since I had very little recollection of what had gone on during the night. But I confirmed that the telephone calls hadn't been about my patient at all, and that I had inadvertently treated a patient I had never seen or heard of before.

Of course, I went to see the twenty-six-year-old patient the next morning. The onset of her coma had been associated with fatigue, weakness, and abdominal pain as well as headache. She then became confused, with disorientation and a loss of vital memory functions before she went into stupor, and was brought into the University Hospital with Kussmaul breathing, a peculiar kind of breathing characteristic of patients in diabetic coma. When I saw her she still seemed fatigued and weak, but her confusion had disappeared and her vital memory had returned to the extent that she knew where she was and what was happening to her.

The lesson to be drawn here is that persons with diabetes who are having memory or mental difficulties should consult their physicians immediately for testing and corrective treatment because these symptoms often indicate a medical problem.

Low Blood Sugar

I'm sure that at some point you have "pigged out" on candy, ice cream, or rich desserts, only to find a couple of hours later that you felt fatigued and even tremulous. You may have suffered an insulin rebound effect from taking too much sugar, which results not in high blood sugar but just the opposite — low blood sugar, or hypoglycemia.

A severe form of this syndrome occurs in people with insulin-secreting tumors of the pancreas, but low blood sugar is also seen in those facing intense stress who are also insulin hypersecreters. In one study a series of medical students had their blood sugar levels taken before and then two hours into an important examination. A surprising number of them had depressed blood sugars. In other words, at a time when they needed their mental resources most, many of them felt weak, tremulous, and had abdominal pain — not a good combination for the best results on an exam.

Harry was a thirty-six-year-old medical student who had such symptoms; glucose tolerance tests showed that his blood sugar went down to very low levels. He went to get a physical examination when he found that his performance was deteriorating and his ability to remember key facts in the clinical cases he was handling had fallen to unacceptable levels.

A test for tumor of the pancreas luckily came back negative. His physician, a gastroenterologist (that is, a doctor specializing in treating diseases of the gastrointestinal tract), decided to give him special medications. He also thought he would try a change in Harry's diet.

First, Harry was taken off all simple sugars: no more sweet desserts, ice cream, or candy. His sources of carbohydrate were limited to starchy foods such as cereals, vegetables, potatoes, and bread. He was allowed to eat a fair amount of protein, especially chicken, turkey, and fish, and he had small meals more frequently dispersed during the day. One of the snacks he enjoyed was peanut butter. Peanut oil contains a substantial amount of mono-unsaturated fatty acids, a relatively harmless kind of fat. This fat did two things to aid Harry's problem: first, it slowed the emptying of his stomach, and second, it made the supply of nutrients in Harry's blood, and in turn to his brain, more evenly distributed, so that an excessive amount of insulin was not secreted.

It is important to recognize and treat hypoglycemia because, in its extreme form, it can cause not only confusion but also epileptic convulsions, postconvulsion stupor, and finally a prolonged state of unconsciousness. If the blood sugar goes down to 30 mg per 100 cc's, confusion, disorientation, and loss of vital memory are all very severe, and it is at this point that epileptic seizures may occur. If the blood sugar goes down to 10 mg per 100 cc's, a profound loss of consciousness results which may produce irreversible damage to the brain. Fortunately, most of us who suffer low levels of blood sugar don't have these severe problems or display such alarming symptoms. We may become nauseated and somewhat tremulous and apprehensive, and our abilities to do complicated intellectual functions, including those that require good recent memory for new learning, are impaired.

If you suspect you have any of these symptoms, see your doctor because the implications of low blood glucose can be verified or disproved by blood tests. Blood sugar levels can be taken after fasting, then a measured amount of glucose is usually taken by mouth and blood sugar tests repeated at 30, 60, 90, 120, 180, and occasionally 240 minutes. Insulin levels can also be determined. If these tests are abnormal, you should seek the attention of a doctor who specializes in blood sugar problems to determine the precise cause. For most people an imbalance in blood sugar is minor and not life-threatening, and the symptoms can often be completely eradicated by changing the diet, as in Harry's case.

Oxygen and Memory Loss

The reduced oxygen supply to the brain in persons with severe anemia or heart or lung disease can cause memory loss. Brain cells, of course, need oxygen. A constant supply of oxygen depends on normal functioning of the heart, and a heart that is failing may not be able to pump blood at the proper rate to supply nutrients and oxygen to the brain. Also, if the blood vessels to the brain are partially occluded or clogged by arteriosclerosis, the amount of blood and therefore oxygen reaching the brain may be insufficient. But even if the heart is working perfectly and the blood vessels are clear, oxygen may be diminished because of lung disease in which too little oxygen is exchanged at the lung capillaries and thus not enough is supplied to support normal function of brain cells. When the lungs are working normally and enough oxygen is delivered into the blood, the oxygen must still be picked up by the hemoglobin, a blood compound containing iron, in the red blood cells. Lack of iron can produce iron deficiency anemia, which can be so severe that an insufficient amount of oxygen is carried to the brain.

Timothy was a forty-three-year-old iron worker who had suffered a head injury at work. He wasn't knocked unconscious and didn't lose his memory when he was injured, but afterward he had great difficulty carrying out his normal functions, was easily fatigued, and couldn't think. His memory abilities, particularly his vital memory functions, were impaired. Timothy's doctors thought that his symptoms were related to his head injury. But when I reviewed his case, more than five years after his accident, it didn't seem to me that Timothy's disabilities all stemmed from a trivial head injury.

I came to this conclusion when I looked over his medical

chart in detail, including records dating from before the injury. At one time he had gone to a doctor claiming to be lightheaded, easily fatigued, and lacking in energy — the same complaints he had after the injury. He had even had a neuropsychological examination, one that was difficult to interpret. His mental functions, and particularly his memory functions, had deteriorated greatly after several hours of testing. The thing no one seemed to pick up on was his severe iron deficiency anemia, a problem that explained both his present symptoms and the abnormalities on his earlier neuropsychological tests.

The lowest limit of the normal range for serum iron is 50. Timothy's was 5, and his hemoglobin was also very low. No wonder he felt lightheaded and weak and fatigued easily. No wonder he had memory failure and failure of mental function. The repeated blood studies, in spite of the fact that he was given supplemental iron, never came back to normal. It was my opinion that a lack of oxygen going to his brain had caused his mental problems. The heme component of the hemoglobin molecule lacked enough iron to hook the oxygen on to.

Timothy was trying to get a sizable settlement for his head injury from an insurance company, but I recommended that before any settlement was made he receive much more adequate treatment for his anemia. This wasn't as easy as it sounds. An iron-rich diet did not bring his serum iron level back to normal, and an extensive series of medical examinations revealed no reason for an extraordinary loss of iron (as, for example, through blood in the stools). Finally, when large amounts of supplementary iron were given, Timothy's serum iron gratifyingly increased to within the normal range, improving his ability to resist fatigue and somewhat restoring his memory and intellectual functions as well.

Of course, oxygen in the blood can also be decreased by any kind of lung disease, such as pneumonia, chronic obstructive lung disease, and lung cancer — diseases often associated with cigarette smoking. Even continual cigarette smoking without obvious lung disease can reduce the amount of oxygen in the blood because of gases inhaled in the cigarette smoke, including carbon gases. It is not surprising, then, when a chronic smoker with lung infection and a smoker's cough exhibits lips and fingernails that are blue or cyanotic and is unable to carry out simple mental tasks because not enough oxygen is going to his brain cells.

Infections that result in a backup of fluids into the lungs — pneumonia, bronchitis, and disorders such as emphysema and congestive heart failure — can interfere with the exchange of oxygen, including the oxygenation of the blood running through the lung capillaries. There is very little that persons with this problem can do to help themselves. Deep breathing, for example, only causes carbon dioxide to be blown off, thereby producing dizziness.

Raising the amount of oxygen in inspired air increases oxygen concentration in the lung capillaries and thus the amount of oxygen going to the brain. But doing so means that an individual must be in an oxygen tent or have a nasal catheter in place through which a continuous flow of oxygen gas is bubbling.

The important factor with lung disease or bronchial tube infections is proper treatment. Sometimes what is required is antibiotic therapy to rid the lungs of infection. At other times the ability of the lungs and bronchial tubes to eliminate secretions that partially or completely plug parts of the respiratory system must be improved. Sometimes surgical treatment is necessary.

The combination of iron deficiency anemia and lung disease may reduce the oxygen level in the brain more sharply than either disease alone, and it is more apt to produce symptoms of reduced memory and mental ability than either disease alone. Of course, both conditions, the lung disease and the anemia, must be treated effectively to reverse memory loss and mental symptoms.

Prevention of Lung Disease

An even more important principle is that of lung disease prevention. Such prevention can be effected by improved working conditions for those involved in some aspects of mining, cotton processing, and other work that can damage the lungs. Avoiding active or passive cigarette smoke is also extremely important. Moreover, asthma must be treated promptly whenever it occurs so that the consequences of chronic lung disease can be avoided, and infections of the pharynx and nasopharynx which might spread into the lower respiratory system must be treated.

In my previous book, *Brain Power,* I gave the example of my old barber who had a smoker's cough and blue fingernails. He kept cutting the hair on one side of my head again and again, ignoring the side left uncut. It's not only barbers who have such problems. I've seen trial lawyers who were heavy smokers sitting in the same kind of dazed condition. And yes, I've even seen physicians with this problem.

An Overview

Vital memory and proper brain function depend on a normal supply of oxygen and glucose being delivered to brain cells through the arteries going to the brain. If the brain is deprived of oxygen for more than a few minutes at normal temperature, irreversible changes can occur in the inner parts of the temporal lobes. In other words, brain cells in the hippocampus, an area that is related to the laying down of new memories, may die.

Similarly, prolonged and deep hypoglycemia, that is, a severely depressed level of blood sugar, may result in convulsions. (Many years ago severe mental illness was treated by artificially producing convulsions through the injection of insulin, which brought about proportionally low levels of blood sugar.) Again, such convulsions cause scarring in the depths of the brain, including the hippocampus, and often resulted in a loss of vital memory.

Most problems related to a lack of sugar or of oxygen going to the brain can be readily treated and reversed. The important thing is to recognize the problem, find its source, and correct it promptly. Correction can mean changing one's diet, having lung problems treated, completely avoiding cigarette smoke, or having severe anemia treated. Whatever treatment measures are necessary, they usually produce a dramatic improvement, including an improvement in memory and brain function, in a relatively short time.

Vital Memory Points to Remember

1. The brain's major fuel is glucose, which must be supplied within certain finite limits for optimal brain and memory functions.
2. Extreme forms of hypoglycemia can cause confusion and epileptic convulsions.
3. Anemia can cause a loss of mental function and vital memory.
4. Cigarette smoking is the most common cause of low oxygen levels in the blood.

12

Thyroid Dysfunction and Memory Loss

Hormonal Balance

WHAT DO YOU THINK of when someone talks about hormones? You most likely don't think of memory loss. Indeed, when the body's hormones are in proper balance there's no danger of their producing memory loss. But if they're out of kilter they can alter the brain's metabolism and chemical environment, which in turn can change brain function for the worse.

You should understand something about hormonal imbalance because these abnormalities can be treated and reversed. Before I describe how hormonal imbalance can produce memory loss, however, you may need a little background on how hormones work and why they're important. Briefly, the brain is extremely dependent on the other organ systems of the body in order to function properly. Hormones secreted by the endocrine glands play an essential role in the process of maintaining homeostasis — keeping the brain's environment balanced.

The master gland that controls many hormones in the body is the pituitary, which is situated at the base of the skull in a little hollow of bone called the Turkish saddle. It is intimately connected with the hypothalamus, which controls fight or flight behavior, proper water balance, body temperature, and natural sleep patterns.

In conjunction with the pineal gland, these tissues regulate the rhythms of the body — not only the wake-sleep cycles but also such patterns as the daily and hourly variations in electrolytes, alterations in the level of clotting factors in the blood, changes in body temperature, and even some emotional changes. These hourly biological changes are called circadian rhythms.

Through various feedback mechanisms, the pituitary also controls the hormonal secretions of other endocrine glands throughout the body. These include the cortex of the adrenal gland, which secretes the steroid hormones; the islands of Langerhans in the pancreas, which secrete insulin (essential for the metabolism of sugar); the parathyroid glands, which control the concentration of calcium in the blood; and the thyroid gland, which controls the rate of metabolism in the body. The pituitary also controls the male testes, which secrete testosterone, and the female ovaries, which secrete estrogen compounds and progesterone.

Each of these hormones has an effect on brain function and memory, but one of the most common hormonal problems (aside from insulin–blood sugar variations) is brought on by decreased levels of thyroid hormone. While small deviations from the normal concentration of thyroid hormone can produce mild changes in brain function, severe memory loss is seen in full-blown cases of hypothyroidism.

Hypothyroidism

One afternoon late in 1989, after I had completed rounds with the neurology residents at a large urban hospital, one of them took me aside and asked me if I wanted to see Oscar, the residents' latest prize patient. He confided that they had just rescued Oscar, a fifty-six-year-old insurance underwriter, from one of the general medical services, which saw him as only another degenerate alcoholic. (The medical service had asked for a neurological consultation since the toxic screen was normal and there was no history of alcoholism.)

Oscar looked like an alcoholic in almost every way. He was disheveled and hadn't shaved or bathed in a long time. He was sluggish in his movements and spent a lot of time just staring at the wall. He wasn't able to give a good account of himself because his memory processes were so slowed.

Blood studies showed that Oscar had severe hypothyroidism — that is, a lack of thyroid hormone secretions. When I saw him he had been cleaned and shaved and had already started treatment with thyroid hormone, but his mental processes were still extremely sluggish. Recent-memory testing showed that he could not remember any of three unrelated objects after a period of two and a half to three minutes, and his recollection of the weeks and months preceding his hospitalization proved to be incomplete and inaccurate. But I was certain his memory problems were reversible, and indeed, with persistent and effective treatment Oscar returned to normal health. A more accurate history taken once he had recovered indicated that he was not, in fact, an alcoholic. It's important to keep in mind, however, that the clinical picture produced by hypothyroidism is easy to misdiagnose as alcoholism, depression, or even Alzheimer's disease, particularly among the elderly, whose physicians often tell the patients' relatives that their gradual mental failure is to be expected — "There's nothing to do about it, it's just old age."

I've seen people similar to Oscar who had been misdiagnosed for many months in nursing homes. One such person benefited from a lecture my colleague, Tom Sabin, gave to a group of nursing home doctors. A doctor who heard Tom's lecture decided he'd test out some of his alleged Alzheimer's patients, and sure enough he found one who was suffering instead from hypothyroidism. The misdiagnosed man responded remarkably well to thyroid hormone. Within several months he had left the nursing home and moved to a rest home, where he was able to take complete charge of his daily activities — dressing, feeding himself, setting his own schedule, and even going out by himself.

Hyperthyroidism Leading to Hypothyroidism

The first case of hypothyroidism, mental deterioration, and memory loss I saw as an intern in 1947 resulted from surgical treatment rather than spontaneous disease causing destruction or malfunction of the thyroid gland. The patient was a forty-seven-year-old bakery clerk named Gloria, who initially had a severe case of hyperthyroidism, characterized by bulging eyes, agitation, irritability, and apprehension. She sometimes became manic and talked a blue streak, interrupted by sudden mood swings and weeping.

In treating her hyperthyroidism, Gloria's surgeon had removed so much of her thyroid gland that what remained did not produce an adequate amount of thyroid hormone. She went from being hyperirritable to being dull, listless, and drowsy. Her speech became somewhat slurred, and her intellectual processes deteriorated because her memory functions were so slowed. She couldn't concentrate, and thus no new memories were acquired, and she had difficulty retrieving old memories from her memory bank. In other words, her thyroid surgery had transformed her from hyperthyroidism to profound hypothyroidism.

I'd like to be able to tell you that the cause of Gloria's problem was immediately understood since it was of course known that she had had much of her thyroid removed. But forty-five years ago this didn't happen, and she became demented before the true nature of her problem was discovered and she was put on thyroid hormone. Even so, treatment did finally reverse her abnormal mental syndrome.

135

Hypothyroidism can occur without a large portion of the thyroid gland having been surgically removed. Ken, an eighty-two-year-old retired bank examiner, had a nodule removed from his thyroid which left most of the gland intact. He seemed to be functioning normally and went for his regular exercise, followed by a steam bath. He couldn't tolerate the steam, however, and he fainted. When he recovered consciousness he wasn't able to function at his previous level, and his doctor thought that he either had had a stroke or was getting Alzheimer's disease, with apathy and memory loss.

Ken subsequently developed an intestinal obstruction, and when he went into a hospital to have this problem surgically corrected it was discovered that his thyroid was underactive. Treatment with thyroid hormone restored him, even at age eighty-two, to normal mental activity. The moral to this story is that anyone who has had thyroid surgery or thyroid dysfunction in the past should have repeated tests of thyroid function to detect and treat abnormalities early so that the difficulties Ken and Gloria encountered can be avoided.

No one should be diagnosed as having Alzheimer's disease before a complete blood and urine evaluation is made by appropriate laboratory studies. Chemical analysis of the blood should always include a thorough check of thyroid function as well as measures of the effectiveness of the liver, the kidneys, and the other endocrine glands as well. Today the dementia and memory loss produced by abnormalities of the thyroid, adrenal cortex, insulin-secreting glands in the pancreas, parathyroid, and pituitary are too easy to diagnose and treat to allow any of them to cause memory loss and mental deterioration.

This is especially true of the hypersecretion of insulin, which depresses the blood sugar, whether the hypersecretion is caused by a pancreatic tumor, emotional lability, or excessive intake of sugar with an insulin rebound. Low blood sugar can readily be identified by blood tests, and treatment may involve only an adjustment in the diet to reverse memory impairment.

Brain functions and especially memory are very susceptible to changes in hormonal levels. And, of course, memory loss always impairs new learning. As a corollary, I believe that people with learning problems should have medical evaluations, including blood tests, to gauge hormonal levels accurately.

Vital Memory Points to Remember

1. Hypothyroidism (a lack of thyroid hormone) can produce clinical symptoms resembling those of alcoholism or even Alzheimer's disease.
2. Hyperthyroidism (too much thyroid hormone) can cause a range of symptoms, including a lack of concentration and hyperdistractibility with secondary memory loss.

Diseases and Injuries That Cause Memory Loss

WHAT IMAGES are conjured up in your mind when you hear of people who have something wrong with their brains? Do you envision a person who acts crazy or stupid, someone who is losing intellectual capacity, or is unable to function, an individual who is comatose or delirious?

Certainly severe problems can afflict the brain, with very undesirable consequences. But remember also that brain sciences have made fantastic progress in the last three decades, in both the diagnosis and treatment of brain diseases and injuries. When pinpointed early, the causes of brain symptoms, especially memory loss, can in many cases be reversed. This fact is important for you to know because many people, when faced with the symptoms of memory loss, become quite depressed. Their first thought is that, like their fathers or grandmothers before them, they've got Alzheimer's disease, that everything is lost, and that there's nothing that can be done for them. Fortunately, that's not true in the vast majority of cases.

After you've read about the various problems described in Part IV you'll begin to see that many different conditions can cause memory loss, that many of them are treatable, and that memory loss is often reversible. It's also good to keep in mind that even people with degenerative brain disease, such as Alzheimer's disease, may have other disorders (like depression, brain poisoning with various drugs or alcohol, malnutrition, or electrolyte imbalance) superimposed on their problem which make the memory loss much worse than it needs to be. Especially in the beginning stages of Alzheimer's, the prevention of or treatment of depression, brain poisoning, malnutrition, or some of the other problems detailed in this part can improve patients' clinical condition and reverse much of their memory loss.

We don't yet have a cure for Alzheimer's, but I do think it's important never to give up hope. Medical research is now being focused on the problems of degenerative brain disease, and they are soluble. It's simply a matter of time and money being applied to research that will ultimately discover the prevention and cure of these diseases. In the meantime, we must give the victims of Alzheimer's and other degenerative brain diseases the best possible treatment. The fewer medical complications they have, the longer they'll be able to live active, full, and interesting lives.

13

Brain Infections That Cause Memory Loss

WHEN WE CONSIDER brain infections that cause memory loss, we're looking at a chapter in medical history which has achieved some amazing triumphs. Many brain infections are completely treatable and curable, and there is hope that rapid progress will be made in conquering those infections, like AIDS, that are not curable at the present time.

Seventy years ago one of the leading causes of memory loss dementia and, indeed, insanity was syphilis of the brain. Now the overwhelming majority of patients with this affliction can be cured by massive doses of penicillin. Newer antibiotics can even cure some brain abscesses that previously had to be drained surgically. Infections caused by bacteria are most readily treated with antibiotics. But even some viral infections can be controlled by antiviral medications if they are given in time. This proved to be true in the case of Hector, a fifty-three-year-old plumber from Boston.

One Sunday about twelve years ago I was called in to a local hospital to do a brain biopsy on Hector, who had a progressive infection of his brain with bizarre changes in personality and severe distortions in memory. Special tests of the brain showed swelling of both temporal lobes, and tests of the blood and spinal fluid gave evidence of infection. As

Hector became more and more ill he had spells of delirium. A tentative diagnosis was made of herpes infection of the brain, so-called herpes encephalitis. This viral encephalitis tends to produce swelling of the temporal lobes and is associated with sudden, rapid changes in personality and severe distortions in brain function, including memory.

An experimental drug was then available which was at least partially effective in arresting herpes infection, but it was also quite toxic. Rather than give a drug that might prove to be inappropriate if the diagnosis was wrong and was in any case potentially lethal, brain biopsies were routinely required before the drug's administration so that the tissue could be cultured and a positive diagnosis of herpes infection of the brain confirmed.

Once the biopsy of Hector's brain had been done, the doctors who supervised the making of viral cultures expected to have a positive culture within twenty-four hours, and certainly within forty-eight. After two days had passed and the culture was still negative, they realized they might not be dealing with a herpes infection of the brain at all, but rather with a disease called Jacob Creutzfeld's syndrome. This dreaded but extremely rare disease produces a rapid onset of dementia and loss of brain function. Absolutely no treatment for it exists. The peculiar organism, the prion, that causes the disease is very resistant to the usual methods of sterilization, and one of the few agents that is effective in sterilizing surgical instruments — that is, that will kill the organism — is chlorine bleach in concentrated solution. The suspicion that Hector's symptoms indicated Jacob Creutzfeld's syndrome put the scrub nurses who had assisted with the biopsy in a panic because the sterile gloves they had worn had holes in them, and moreover one of them had a wound on her hand and was convinced that this fearsome organism had entered her body.

Finally, after ninety-six hours had passed, a positive diagnosis of herpes encephalitis was confirmed by Hector's culture, and the panic in the nursing staff abated. In the meantime, however, all surgical instruments were soaked in bleach solution, with the unhappy outcome of destroying some of the more delicate ones. The Jacob Creutzfeld's scare in the operating room cost the hospital around $3,500 to replace these instruments. But Hector's case ended better: the new drugs against herpes encephalitis were effective, and Hector made a nice recovery, reverting to his normal personality and improved recent-memory function.

Brain infections can be caused by bacteria, fungi, protozoans, or viruses. They may be generalized in the brain, producing a disease like sleeping sickness, or they can be localized in one part of the brain. If the local infection is walled off by reactive tissue, it will form an abscess and has to be treated surgically by drainage or removal. Infections can invade the brain from infected nasal sinuses or mastoids or from infections in the blood. No matter how it occurs, any infection of the brain is a serious medical problem.

Infections of the entire brain, such as in encephalitis, may be closely related to infections of the tissues covering the brain, the meninges. These infections, called meningitis, are often characterized by high fever, headaches, and a stiff neck. If the meningeal infection spreads to the brain tissue, it may irritate brain cells enough to cause epileptic seizures. A correct diagnosis in cases of this kind is extremely important. If meningitis is suspected, a careful spinal puncture should be carried out to analyze the spinal fluid. With infants and young children especially, high fever alone, without any infection of the brain or spinal fluid, can trigger an epileptic convulsion in patients whose threshold for epileptic seizures is decreased.

Identifying Brain Infections

Many kinds of brain infection produce changes in personality and decrease memory abilities, including infections that are secondary to such viral diseases as measles. Some viral infections — herpes for instance — tend to localize in structures related to memory function, like the temporal lobes. This localization also occurs with the virus that causes rabies, which produces characteristic changes in the hippocampus as well as the most severe changes in personality and behavior. Its very name — in French, *rage;* in Italian, *rabia;* and in German, *wut* — means "madness" or "rage."

The recognition of acute brain infections is usually not difficult. The patient becomes very ill with fever, and noticeable changes in personality and behavior gradually occur. The person will also complain of severe headaches and frequently exhibit epileptic convulsions.

To diagnose the cause of the problem, a general physical examination should be performed, including a neurological evaluation. Observation of the likely places where infection can start — the paranasal sinuses, mastoids, lungs, or heart (in individuals who have heart disease, which allows the shunting of infectious material through abnormal openings into the circulation of the brain) — aids in recognizing the sites of brain infection. Blood tests, both to make cultures and to see how the white blood cells are responding to the infection, are helpful. The most important test is usually a spinal puncture, which allows direct culture of the spinal fluid, and microscopic examination to see if any organisms can be recognized. Also, it's then possible to look at the cells in the spinal fluid and find whether or not spinal fluid chemistries are normal.

Therapies for Brain Infections

Once an infection has been diagnosed, specific therapies are undertaken in the most vigorous fashion. If the infection

144

is bacterial, the appropriate antibiotic or combination of antibiotics must be administered promptly. If the infection is
viral, antiviral medications can be given, although it should
be pointed out that some viral agents don't respond well to
medications, and moreover, some of the medications used to
treat viral infections are themselves toxic and must be given
with great care. Specific agents also exist to treat infections by
spirochetes, as well as fungi.

I'd like to insert a word of caution here about the unre-
stricted use of spinal puncture before a complete neurological
examination is done, including an ophthalmoscopic examination through the eyeball of the optic nerve head. If the
optic disc is swollen, it may mean that there is increased
pressure in the head, in which case a CAT scan or MRI
examination of the brain should be performed before any
spinal fluid is obtained by a spinal puncture. This routine
serves as a precaution so that if a localized mass is present in
the brain, such as a brain abscess, a protective cushion of
spinal fluid will not be removed by a spinal puncture, allowing a portion of the brain mass to herniate against the brain
stem.

Brain Abscesses

An abscess or localized brain infection is common
enough that we should always keep the possibility in mind,
even in persons who seem to exhibit the more generalized
signs of brain infection. Most abscesses have to be evacuated
and drained surgically or completely excised; only a few in
the earliest stages can be successfully treated by massive
antibiotic therapy.

Robert, twenty, a truck driver, was a muscular man who
came to the hospital with a draining right ear and an infection
of his middle ear and mastoid. He was immediately admitted
when his neck became very stiff and he had an epileptic seizure. Following treatment, Robert recovered from the seizure,

but he continued to have an intermittent spiking temperature and was confused and irrational at times. He also had a loss of recent memory. Over the course of several weeks, his vital memory deteriorated to the point that he recklessly broke social taboos by urinating in his bed and repeatedly masturbating in the open ward. He was belligerent as well, striking out at anyone who tried to examine or treat him.

Radio-opaque dye was injected into the major artery going to Robert's brain on the side of his draining ear, and x rays were taken as the dye traveled through the blood vessels of his brain. These x rays showed that Robert had a large abscess in the front end of his temporal lobe. Once the abscess was excised surgically his symptoms began to abate. The surgical excision was accompanied by effective treatment with antibiotics, which killed the offending bacterial organisms. Not only did Robert get back his vital memory, but his entire mental function soon returned to normal.

Physicians don't always do a spinal puncture in evaluating patients whose memory faculties and intellectual abilities are deteriorating, but perhaps they should, as the case of Jeremy, a sixty-three-year-old middle school teacher, illustrates. Jeremy had suffered a progressive loss of memory and was thought to be in the beginning stages of Alzheimer's disease. In the hospital, the results of all blood and urine tests, a medical examination, the CAT scan of his brain, and a brain wave test were within normal limits. He was discharged, yet his mental decline continued. Jeremy had to come to the hospital a second time before a lumbar puncture was carried out. The subsequent examination of his spinal fluid showed that it contained fungi and that he had a fungal infection around the base of his brain. The treatment of this infection brought some improvement, but he had residual memory loss that prevented him from being fully effective as a teacher, and he had to retire. His retirement would have been unnecessary if his problem had been diagnosed earlier.

Fungal infections of the brain and meninges are uncommon, but they can occur in anyone with an immune system deficiency, as in patients with AIDS. It is important to treat these infections early, and a spinal fluid exam should be done in every case of dementia which cannot be explained by routine testing.

Syphilitic Brain Infection

Two diseases that are sexually transmitted or spread through blood contact can produce late-onset infections of the brain, with resultant loss of memory and other intellectual functions. These only superficially similar diseases are syphilis and AIDS. Produced by a spirochete called treponema, syphilis progresses in three distinct phases: first, the primary chancre appears, usually on the genitals; a secondary outbreak of lesions can be in the mouth; finally, after five, ten, fifteen, even twenty years or more, an infection of the brain or of the great vessels of the heart occurs. Although it is relatively uncommon today, syphilis of the brain used to fill the insane asylums and state mental hospitals with infected patients in the early part of this century.

Charlie, who was in the wholesale grocery business, was a patient of my father's who contracted syphilis about twenty years before I saw him. During my father's time, of course, there was no such thing as penicillin, and my father treated Charlie with drugs compounded from arsenic and with bismuth, and he gave him injections over a period of four or five years in the hope of eradicating the infection. My father was assiduous in checking for any problems in his patient's heart vessels, but Charlie didn't show signs of heart trouble, nor did he have another common complication of syphilis, tabes dorsalis, a syphilitic infection of the spinal cord. He did, however, develop syphilis of the brain.

I saw Charlie after my father died, when Charlie was sixty-seven years old. He had begun to have unusual changes in

his moods, swinging from depression to unpredictable out-
breaks of rage. He had always been a rather mild-mannered
individual, and his sister, who lived with him, became
deathly frightened when he started to threaten her. He also
told me that he was having difficulty with his memory, and
that his intellectual abilities had declined so that he was afraid
he was making mistakes in his business.

Since my father's old records showed that many years before Charlie had had syphilis, I drew some blood to test for
syphilis. But although the blood test was negative, Charlie's
symptoms persisted. Just to be on the safe side, I decided to
do a spinal puncture. I drew some spinal fluid and sent it to
the state laboratory. Unlike the blood sample, the spinal fluid
proved to be positive for syphilis, and I started treating Charlie with what was then a new drug, penicillin.

Oddly enough, a lot of doctors at first didn't have much
confidence in penicillin for the treatment of syphilis, although of course over time it proved to be of immense value.
Eventually Charlie's mental problems and his failing memory
improved quite dramatically, and repeated examinations of
his spinal fluid showed that he was free from syphilitic infection.

AIDS and Memory Loss

Autoimmune deficiency syndrome attacks the ability of
the body's immune system to ward off disease, but it can also
cause infections of the brain. At first we didn't realize that the
brain, along with the immune system, is a primary target for
the AIDS virus because the attack on the immune system
produces all sorts of bizarre infections, some of which metastasize to the brain. It also makes patients susceptible to certain tumors or cancers, which invade the brain, and causes
brain hemorrhages in some patients. Moreover, an individual
infected with the AIDS virus can get a transient infection of
the meninges, the tissues around the brain, after which the

person may be asymptomatic for months or even years.

Researchers originally believed that all these brain problems were secondary to the assault on the immune system. However, AIDS patients often seemed unusually depressed and apathetic, and they had a noticeable reduction in intellectual ability and recent memory without showing focal lesions in the brain. We learned that these symptoms were due not to depression, but to an infestation of the brain by the AIDS virus itself which blocked the action of certain essential neurotransmitters.

Kevin was a skillful anesthesiologist at one of the hospitals where I worked. He became increasingly worried when some of his homosexual contacts developed clinical symptoms of AIDS. Then a blood test showed that he himself was positive for the AIDS virus. Initially Kevin became somewhat depressed and couldn't function very well. A CAT scan revealed brain atrophy, particularly in the front part of his brain.

Unhappily for Kevin, AZT had not yet been developed as a treatment for AIDS. His mental deterioration progressed rapidly, and subsequent CAT scans showed continuing alarming shrinkage of his brain. Kevin committed suicide less than a year before AZT became available for treating AIDS. Only ten months after Kevin's suicide, in fact, we used AZT in treating a twenty-seven-year-old Haitian nurse who had an AIDS infection of the brain, dementia, and loss of recent memory, and she experienced a remarkable return of her intellectual abilities. Of course, AZT is not a cure for AIDS, and the improvement is temporary. Nevertheless, the improvement may last for several years with effective continued treatment.

What to Look For in Brain Infections and How to Get Help

Brain infections can produce adverse changes in mental abilities, with major decreases in recent and other aspects of vital memory, through direct infestation of the brain, through consequent epileptic seizures, or through the delirium associated with infection. Overwhelming acute brain infections are easily diagnosed, but as I mentioned earlier, some persons with smoldering brain infections may be misdiagnosed as having dementia or even depression. One physician prescribed electroshock treatments for a very apathetic seamstress who was misdiagnosed as suffering from depression. When we did a spinal tap, our examination of her spinal fluid showed that she had bacterial meningitis, which was successfully treated with antibiotics.

The same rules for diagnosing other causes of memory loss — obtaining a good history and making thorough physical and laboratory examinations — also hold in diagnosing brain infection. Because some infections, if untreated, have a rapid and even fatal course, it is necessary to diagnose them with great dispatch.

With chronic infections, or those that progress slowly over weeks or months, we must exercise greater vigilance and suspicion, especially when these infections invade the inner portions of the temporal lobes, interfering with the memory process. The mood changes caused by some chronic infections mimic psychiatric problems and dementia. Patients are misdiagnosed as being severely depressed when, in fact, their problem is caused by direct brain infection. Diagnostic caution is especially called for in cases of tertiary syphilis as well as in some of the newer threats we all face, such as AIDS. Finally, we must not rule out brain infections such as syphilis as the cause of dementia and memory loss in elderly patients. Again, a spinal fluid examination may be critical in confirming the diagnosis.

The most important factor to consider with respect to brain infections is their prevention. Childhood immunization for measles also obviously prevents the complication of measles encephalitis. Prompt treatment of infections in other parts of the body, such as mastoid and sinus infections, will avert their spread to the brain. In areas of endemic encephalitis, avoiding mosquito bites by not going out at night, when mosquitoes are abundant, or using copious amounts of mosquito repellants is also wise. As far as diseases like AIDS and syphilis are concerned, avoiding sexual promiscuity and, in the former case, avoiding the sharing of needles among intravenous drug users are critical in preventing brain infection.

As fast as we develop new antibiotics and methods of immunization, ever more exotic infectious agents seem to appear on the medical scene. Some of these can be found in hospital settings, and even in blood banks. Every area of medical practice — hospitals, clinics, blood banks — must therefore continue to use the most scrupulous care to avoid transmitting infectious agents, particularly those that can cause damage to our vital memory functions.

Vital Memory Points to Remember

1. Brain infections can be caused by bacteria, fungi, protozoans, and viruses, all of which can produce memory loss.
2. A brain abscess is a localized brain infection that can result in confusion, irritability, memory loss, seizures, and signs of increased pressure in the brain.
3. Sexually transmitted diseases and diseases carried by blood, including AIDS, produce a variety of brain infections, all of which can cause memory loss.

14

Closed-Head Injuries and Memory Loss

IN MY MEDICAL PRACTICE I've seen literally hundreds of patients with closed-head injuries that resulted in mild to severe loss of memory. The vast majority of these injuries were caused by automobile collisions. Because some people walk away from car crashes without realizing how badly they've been injured, it sometimes takes weeks before the resulting loss of brain function is reported. Quite often it is not even the victim but rather a close friend or relative who recognizes the loss of memory function and encourages the patient to seek medical treatment. Indeed, closed-head injuries may produce such a prolonged decline in memory and mental abilities that even the reluctant patient will finally agree that medical treatment is the only viable course of action.

Because the brain is a semigelatinous mass with a cushion of spinal fluid around and within it, suspended on a fountain of blood within the bony box that is the cranium, it can withstand most minor bumps and bruises without ill effect. But any acceleration or deceleration accident whose impact exceeds the elasticity of the brain and the cushioning effect of the spinal fluid will damage the base of the frontal lobes and the tips of the temporal lobes. In addition, if there is twisting or turning of the head, tearing of the axons, the nerve fibers leading impulses away from the brain cells may occur.

The injuries I've just described are different from open-head injuries, in which there is a penetrating wound of the brain. Being hit by a bullet or a baseball bat, for example, causes a depressed fracture of the skull, with bone slivers penetrating the membranes of the brain and actually sticking into the brain itself. Open-head injuries obviously cause brain damage, and often secondary epileptic seizures, because of their direct effect on brain tissue. But the closed-head injury, in which no penetration of the skull occurs, can also wreak destructive effects in the front part of the brain and on the internal fibers of the brain.

The complications of both closed- and open-head injuries are magnified in the elderly. The brains of older persons have fewer brain cells and lesser redundancy, so that any loss of function is less apt to be compensated for by recircuiting through another, uninjured pathway, such as occurs in a younger individual or especially in a child. Also, the smaller volume of the brains of elderly persons makes their brains more susceptible to tears of blood vessels in angular, decelerating brain injuries.

The Three Kinds of Closed-Head Injuries

Closed-head injuries fall into three categories. Major head injuries, which require hospitalization for more than twenty-four hours, result in loss of consciousness or memory for more than twenty to forty minutes and of course produce prolonged loss of brain function. Minor head injuries, treated during a hospital stay of less than twenty-four hours, produce a loss of consciousness or memory for less than twenty minutes. But the fact that a head injury is deemed minor does not make it insignificant. Such trivial head injuries are the kind children often get when they bump their heads. No real injury to the brain itself occurs because the cushioning effect of the spinal fluid and the absorption of the energy of impact by the scalp and skull prevent damage to underlying brain tissue.

Most head injuries (except in the elderly, who are more at risk than the young) are of the trivial variety and need not concern us. It's the so-called minor head injuries that turn out to be not so minor. They are not only associated with memory problems lasting anywhere from four to six weeks, but also with difficulties in social adjustment, marital harmony, and work performance as well as with depression that may endure for many months and even years. When these complications of minor head injuries are superimposed on a heart or liver condition, for example, which many people in their seventies or eighties may have, their effects prove to be minor only in comparison with those of the life-threatening and devastating major head injuries. In addition, even mild head injuries in the elderly can have late complications such as subdural hematomas.

Carlos was a sixty-year-old jazz musician who played various kinds of electric guitars. One night the members of his band finished work late, after public transportation had stopped running, and so Carlos asked one of the band members to drive him home. When he was dropped off he tried to leave the car quickly, but in doing so he accidentally closed the car door on his coat. When the car suddenly accelerated, Carlos was upended and bounced along the highway, on his head, for about twenty-five feet before his anguished cry caused the driver of the car to stop.

Although he was dazed and briefly lost his memory of some of the events that occurred at the time of his injury, examinations at the hospital did not disclose any skull fracture, and Carlos was sent home. Headaches, difficulty with recent memory, inability to plan, a lack of initiative, and a complete disintegration of his work-related activities persisted for some months after his head injury.

When it became obvious that he could no longer perform at his previous level, Carlos sought medical help. A complete neurological evaluation showed some abnormalities in the neuropsychological exam and in the computerized brain wave test. But these were minor compared with the social and functional impairment Carlos suffered. This man was not having seizures and was not an alcohol or drug abuser. I noted that he was clearly depressed, which is common after a minor brain injury. And, of course, depression may have exacerbated his problems with recent memory.

Treatment of the depression, along with large doses of tincture of time, was the prescription that worked in Carlos's case. It took almost two years before he returned to the same level of activity he had engaged in before his head injury, but he did recover fully.

Disability After a Minor Head Injury

The clinical course of chronic disability after a minor head or brain injury is all too common. The patient has objective signs of memory loss which clear up after four to six weeks, but is then left with disabling depression, headache, changes in mood and behavior, difficulty in social interactions, trouble in performing any kind of job, and increasing friction and tension in domestic relationships. From my own experience and reports in the literature on head injuries, I would judge that there may be more than a hundred thousand patients a year who suffer minor head or brain injuries, chiefly in automobile accidents, and whose course is similar to that of Carlos. All too often cases of this sort end up in court, usually because the representatives of insurance companies don't believe that minor head injuries can be so disabling. A small percentage of these patients injure their heads at work, in which case they come up in review before workers' compensation boards. The issue of financial compensation by insurance companies in cases of prolonged disability

155

has been subjected to intense scrutiny. But although the precise cause of disability is often not agreed on, there is no question that such disability stemming from head injuries is genuine. It is not a "compensation neurosis" — that is, a problem with physical symptoms which disappear once a settlement is reached.

Amnesia and Closed-Head Injuries

The immediate consequences of head injury may be retrograde amnesia, in which the victim has difficulty recalling events that preceded the brain injury, or antrograde amnesia, in which the victim blocks out for a matter of minutes to hours, or sometimes even days, the events following a head injury.

That's what happened to Karen, a fifty-seven-year-old instructor, who was sitting in the passenger seat of an automobile struck head-on by a drunken driver speeding in the wrong lane. She was unconscious for a time following the injury and was in the hospital for several weeks. She then began to make a gradual recovery, to the extent that six months later she returned to teaching. Karen then found that her ability to study and teach was compromised, which clearly signaled memory problems since the recent-memory function is central to the acquisition of new information — that is, to learning. Karen had to transfer many of her students to other teachers and dropped down to limited teaching.

She sued the drunken driver, but when the case went to trial, the insurance company covering the other driver minimized Karen's problems, saying that because she was able to teach in a college, she couldn't have suffered major brain injury. It was at this point that we undertook a full evaluation of Karen's case, including neuropsychological and psychodiagnostic tests as well as brain wave studies, neurological

156

examinations, and a CAT scan of the brain. Karen's brain examinations showed a previously unsuspected hole inside her brain which had been caused by the destruction of brain tissue at the time of the accident. This loss of brain tissue resulted in her loss of memory.

Karen's case has two important lessons. First, even patients over fifty who have had major brain injuries may recover a significant amount of their mental abilities, so that inexperienced observers may say that they are completely normal when they are not. And second, even when such recovery takes place, a full neurological evaluation is necessary to pinpoint residual problems. This is important not only in working out programs for future rehabilitation but also in determining the amount of functional loss. When Karen's loss was presented to a jury, she was compensated with over $3 million in damages.

In my experience, neither the patient nor the physician should ever give up hope of recovery after a serious head injury. The mental abilities of one of my patients, a sixty-three-year-old man who had experienced severe intellectual deterioration and memory loss after a major head injury, were significantly restored *five years* after the damage to his brain occurred. Such improvement is more likely in a closed- than in an open-head injury because extreme loss of brain tissue is less common in patients who suffer closed-head injury.

Seat Belts, Air Bags, and Head Injuries

Every year, as many as half a million persons in the United States injure their brains as a result of automobile collisions. Of the fifty thousand or more people who die in automobile accidents, seventy percent of the deaths are due directly to brain injury. Some other victims who survive are so severely brain-injured and have lost so much of their vital memories that they will spend the rest of their lives in chronic care institutions. Many of the others with less serious injuries will substantially recover. Even so, they may have lost some brain function if their injuries have caused a loss of brain tissue, which cannot regenerate.

The clear message from all these facts is the importance of prevention. If every automobile in the United States were equipped with three-point shoulder and lap restraints, plus air bags for every passenger, most of these brain injuries and deaths would be averted. This solution is expensive, of course — but it is even more expensive to care for chronically disabled brain-injured patients who will remain in nursing homes for the rest of their lives. Finally, we must consider more than just the expenditure of money. We also have to think of the waste of human potential and the interruption of useful lives which are a consequence of brain injury. This effect is magnified in the elderly, who tolerate brain injury to a lesser extent than do younger persons.

It is within our power to exert the political and moral persuasion that will reduce or prevent most brain injuries, through an educational campaign directed at the president of the United States and the U.S. Congress. Congress should legislate national safety standards for every car and truck on the road, which would virtually eliminate the occurrence of the majority of serious brain injuries. That such legislation has not yet been passed is a national tragedy.

Vital Memory Points to Remember

1. Closed-head injuries are most often caused by automobile accidents.
2. Even so-called minor head injuries can result in difficulties with mental functioning and memory for months and years.

3. Half a million persons injure their heads as a result of car collisions in the United States each year. One hundred thousand of these injuries are serious.

4. Installation of air bags in cars and use of three-point shoulder restraints would greatly reduce the severity of head injuries sustained in accidents.

15

Epilepsy and Memory Loss

HAVE YOU EVER SEEN someone have an epileptic seizure? Do you think that people who have epilepsy are different from you and me? If you do, you're wrong; anyone, you
and me included, could have a seizure if our brains were
subjected to sufficient injury or toxic exposure. Contrary to
what you may have thought, epilepsy is actually a symptom
rather than a disease, characterized by episodic alterations in
consciousness related to electrical abnormalities in the brain.
Anyone, I would like to reiterate, if given enough brain poisons like alcohol or cocaine, can have an epileptic seizure,
although individuals with a family predisposition to seizures
may have a lower threshold for them than the average
person. And, of course, seizures can be provoked not only
by brain poisons but also by brain tumors, brain injuries,
strokes, and brain infections.

What many people often forget is that epileptic seizures
can be either generalized or localized. There are two kinds of
generalized seizures. The grand mal seizure, the classic major
seizure, is associated with complete loss of consciousness,
breath holding, urinary incontinence, tongue biting, fixed
posture and alternating contraction of the muscles, and ster-

torous breathing (a heavy snoring sound), whereas the petit mal seizure, which is most often seen in children, brings about just small lapses in consciousness.

A localized, or partial, epileptic seizure can start at any area of the brain which is irritated, producing a seizure related to a specific brain structure. A seizure in the motor area, for instance, can cause an epileptic movement in a hand or the side of the mouth; in the sensory area of the brain, it can produce sensations. These partial seizures can become generalized, or they can remain local.

If seizures occur in the emotional or limbic part of the brain, the area associated with the laying down of new memories, they are known as partial complex seizures. These spells can start with the hallucination of a bad smell or bad taste, or a funny feeling in the abdomen. They are succeeded by chewing movements and occasionally automatic behavior — that is, making an inappropriate movement again and again. Partial complex seizures may also develop into generalized seizures. Sometimes just a fragment of the seizure is observable — the "aura" or warning, such as a bad taste or smell, or a blank stare on the face of the patient for just a few moments.

Some of my patients who experienced this kind of seizure became belligerent during and immediately before or after the seizure. But most often belligerence, excessive religiosity, forced writing, and a profound lack of sexual drive were seen between seizures rather than during the episodes themselves. Such changes are rare in epilepsy originating in the nonemotional parts of the brain.

Partial Complex Seizures and Memory Loss

Because limbic or partial complex seizures so often begin in the anterior medial part of the temporal lobes, in close proximity to important parts of the memory circuit, loss of memory is a frequent consequence, one that often manifests itself clinically in periods of confusion. And if an individual has repeated small seizures, loss of memory may be so intense that long-lasting confusion results.

Very occasionally, seizures produce loss of memory for a length of time during which the patient engages in rather complicated but appropriate behavior. Such was the case with Fred, twenty-eight, an ex-marine who had a small shrapnel wound in one of his temporal lobes, the scar of which generated partial complex seizures.

After Fred got out of the Marine Corps on disability, he took a job driving a tractor-trailer between Reno and Los Angeles. He described episodes of having these little blackout spells just outside Reno and coming to his senses as he was nearing the truck depot in Los Angeles. Incredibly, Fred would have no idea of how he got from one place to the other, although on one occasion a relief driver who was with him swore that he did everything perfectly, drove safely, and completed his run on time.

When Fred consulted me about his seizures, he was obviously quite disturbed. Even though we were able to reduce the number of his seizures and the resultant memory loss by the use of antiseizure medication, he quit truck driving and became an electrician: "It was just too nerve-racking," he explained.

Epileptic Seizures in Older Individuals

At times an epileptic seizure may be the first symptom of a problem of the brain needing urgent attention. Generalized seizures are easy to recognize, but partial seizures can too readily be missed, particularly when they occur in an older individual. They may be misdiagnosed as Alzheimer's disease or some other incurable and progressive ailment, or as simply a loss of function with old age. Misdiagnosis is especially regrettable when memory loss, periods of confusion, and seeming dementia are caused by seizures, since they are readily treatable and the memory loss they cause can be reversed.

Epileptic Seizures and Alzheimer's

If seizures occur at all in Alzheimer's disease, they happen very late in the progress of the disorder, when intellectual loss is advanced and recent and remote memory are nil. Seizures usually do not occur early in the course of the disease, and therefore when patients have seizures and their main problem is loss of memory, without any great loss of intellectual capacity, it is quite unlikely that the correct diagnosis is Alzheimer's disease.

Because they abnormally block memory pathways, seizures can produce confusional states and loss of memory without any other brain disease being present. Small, repeated seizures that are difficult to discern can cause long-lasting loss of memory, which is hard to differentiate from memory loss resulting from other causes, such as tiny strokes or the beginning stages of Alzheimer's disease.

Detecting Epileptic Seizures

Finally, you should be aware that some seizures cannot be detected, even by brain wave tests, especially when the seizures occur deep within the brain — such as, for example, near certain sensitive parts of the memory circuits. Partial complex seizures, or minor seizures, may occur in the depths of the brain while surface recordings show normal brain wave activity. This fact makes it all the more difficult to establish a positive and accurate diagnosis, and repeated examinations, including twenty-four-hour brain wave recordings, are often necessary. Even so, these sophisticated examinations may still miss small seizures that disrupt memory function and produce confusion, and patients suspected of having such seizures are therefore sometimes given a therapeutic trial of antiseizure medication.

163

Any past history of brain trauma, brain infection, or childhood or febrile convulsions, or a family history of seizures, should increase your awareness of this possible cause of periods of confusion and memory loss. You should know too that strokes and brain hemorrhages may also produce electrical disturbances and seizures. And, of course, any kind of structural brain abnormality seen on a CAT or MRI scan, such as a brain tumor or arteriovenous malformation, can also generate a seizure disorder. Keep in mind, however, that although structural abnormalities can increase the tendency to have seizures, no matter whether an epileptic seizure or convulsion is generalized or partial, it is a functional disturbance of the brain. Temporary or prolonged memory loss and confusion are frequently the result.

Great advances have been made in the treatment of epilepsy by medication. Tracey Putnam, a neurosurgeon who preceded me at the Boston City Hospital, discovered the effectiveness of Dilantin in preventing seizures in the 1930s. This agent was the first to stop seizures without producing sedation. Partial complex seizures have similarly been helped by the use of another medicine called Tegretol, and attacks of petit mal epilepsy have been reduced in frequency by valproic acid medications. Occasionally, when medications don't work, the surgical removal of an epileptic focus will eliminate seizures. Through reduction or elimination of seizures, the confusion and memory loss that accompany them can also be reversed.

Vital Memory Points to Remember
1. Epilepsy is a symptom, not a disease.
2. If given enough brain poisons, anyone can have an epileptic seizure.
3. Memory loss is common during epileptic seizures.
4. Once diagnosed, memory loss caused by seizures can be restored once the seizures are stopped.

16

Strokes and Memory Loss

YOU MAY HAVE the notion that all patients with strokes are paralyzed and that there's not much you can do for them, but that notion is wrong. The symptoms of some stroke patients can be reversed with treatment. Rehabilitation therapies can improve the condition of many stroke victims and, of course, many strokes can be prevented by reducing fats in the diet and by effectively treating high blood pressure.

There are various kinds of stroke, many of which can bring about memory loss. Not all strokes are the same, and what's more, their treatments are not the same. Major strokes are of two varieties: those related to rupturing of a blood vessel, leading to brain hemorrhage; and those related to the closing off or plugging up of a blood vessel by an embolus or arteriosclerotic occlusion. This shuts off the flow of blood through the vessel, depriving an area of the brain of its blood supply and killing the affected segment of brain tissue. This is called a cerebral infarct.

Major infarcts are announced at times by blindness or paralysis that lasts for a few minutes and then goes away. These temporary strokes, called transient ischemic attacks, are caused by tiny platelet emboli from ulcers in the carotid artery in the neck — or by incomplete closure of the brain's blood vessels. They are often a warning that a major stroke is on the way, and prompt treatment is necessary, such as surgery to remove arteriosclerotic plaques from the diseased carotid artery. The operation, called a carotid endarterectomy, is often effective in preventing further trouble. Even when the source of a stroke is a hemorrhage instead of an infarct, surgical removal of the hemorrhage is often possible, depending on its location and cause.

Multi-Infarct Dementia

Surprisingly, because they are often multiple, small or tiny strokes are a frequent cause of memory loss and intellectual and mood changes, producing a syndrome called multi-infarct dementia. In one variety of this disorder, patients' small blood vessels in their brains are fairly normal but the large blood vessels in their necks, such as the carotids, have blood vessel disease, or the patients may have abnormal areas in the linings of their hearts. These areas are predisposed to clot formation and small clots or parts of clots may break off, forming emboli that travel to the smaller tiny blood vessels of the brain, where they block the vessels and produce small infarcts, or strokes. As can be seen in the case of Hattie, the clinical pattern of these strokes is characteristic.

Hattie was the sixty-seven-year-old matriarch of a large family, and three of her daughters as well as many grandchildren lived with her. She was a God-fearing, hard-working woman who held a full-time job in a factory, kept the family accounts, and was extremely responsible.

One morning Hattie's oldest daughter found her wandering around her bedroom, seemingly dazed and confused. When the daughter told her that she would be late for work, she couldn't seem to focus on the words, and she made no attempt to get dressed. Hattie's daughter called her employer and told him that her mother was sick and couldn't come in — which in itself was unusual since Hattie hadn't missed a day of work in decades. For the next three or four days, although her confusion persisted, she seemed to recover little by little. When a week had passed she seemed ready to get on with her life.

But Hattie's mental powers weren't quite as good as they had been before. She wasn't as alert or as focused. She knew generally what she had to do, but she wasn't the sharp executive who ran the entire family so efficiently. Gradually her daughters took over a fair amount of responsibility. Life went on for another six or seven weeks, and then the same thing happened all over again, except that this time her confusional period and memory loss lasted a little longer and her recovery was even less perfect.

I hear this kind of story often from people with multi-infarct dementia. They have small strokes, often occurring deep inside the brain and in a variable pattern, which reduce recent memory and seem to be progressive. Some victims of this disease are misdiagnosed as having Alzheimer's. And, of course, when they go to their doctors, they're told that there's nothing that can be done for them, and no further investigation of possible causes of their problem is made.

Some researchers think that multi-infarct dementia is always caused by the closing off of very tiny blood vessels in the brain — that is, small arteries. But an astute neuropathologist who did post-mortem examinations on multi-infarct dementia patients who died failed to find much evidence of primary blood vessel disease. He has postulated that sometimes the disease is caused by little clots that break off from the great vessels in the neck which go to the brain, or from the lining of the heart itself, or from a diseased valve of the heart. This theory, if confirmed, has practical significance because medicines (including aspirin) that thin the blood and reduce clotting may prevent the recurrence of this problem. Depending on the site at which the clots originate, surgical treatment may also be helpful.

167

Tests for Diagnosing Multi-Infarct Dementia (Type I)

Anthony, a fifty-seven-year-old ranch worker, had been complaining of feeling faint and having difficulty with recent memory. He went to see a neurosurgeon because an article in the local newspaper had told about some remarkable surgical treatment that helped people with just his symptoms. The article stated that local hardening of the arteries in the great vessels of the neck narrowed the blood vessels to such an extent that a noise resulted as the blood rushed by the area of partial obstruction. It furthermore stated that to screen for this problem, a doctor could put a stethoscope to the patient's neck and would be able to hear the noise of the blood passing through the constricted area.

Besides feeling faint and showing signs of memory failure, Anthony had been hearing a funny noise in one ear. So he looked up the neurosurgeon mentioned in the newspaper article and made an urgent appointment. When the doctor listened at his neck he heard a striking bruit corresponding to the noise Anthony himself heard.

All this took place before the invention of CAT scans and magnetic resonance imaging. The neurosurgeon made extensive x-ray tests, placing a small catheter in the great vessels carrying arterial blood to the brain and injecting these vessels with radio-opaque solutions that could be visualized by x rays as the solution went through the blood vessels. In this way he followed the course of the radio-opaque solution from the base of the neck all the way up to the brain.

Fortunately for Anthony, his partial blockage occurred in only one of his carotid arteries at the point where it branched into the internal and external divisions. Surgical treatment required opening the artery and carefully removing the arteriosclerotic plaque that obstructed the passage, making certain that no little clots broke off and deposited themselves in the brain.

Anthony seemed to be perfectly all right, with good neurological function, in the immediate postoperative period.
But about six hours later he began to feel weakness in one
arm and his lower face, on the side opposite to where the
operation had been performed. The surgeon thought the clot
might have recurred at the site of the operation and that he
might have to go in and remove it. But first he elevated
Anthony's blood pressure, and the partial paralysis disappeared. The doctor had to keep the blood pressure elevated
for about three days, then gradually allowed it to drift back to
normal. Anthony had no further symptoms, and he was able
to go back to work without any problems. More important,
he did not have any episodes of tiny strokes caused by the
breaking off of little clots or groups of platelets from the
diseased artery because the anatomical site that could harbor
clots and potential emboli had been completely removed.

Ultrasound of the heart and of the great blood vessels in
the neck may be helpful in determining which of the possible
sites of embolic strokes is at fault. In addition, x rays following the injection of radio-opaque substances into the blood
stream as well as specialized MRI scans may help locate the
site of the problem in the blood vessels and heart. And of
course today CAT scans and magnetic resonance images of
the brain can establish the clinical diagnosis of multi-infarct
dementia anatomically.

An important message I want to convey is not to take the
diagnosis of Alzheimer's disease as final until a very thorough and accurate history has been taken. If a person with
decreasing memory has had episodes of confusion, with
gradual improvement until the next episode, the problem is
probably not Alzheimer's disease but multi-infarct dementia
produced by these tiny repeated strokes. The great tragedy is
that if this condition is left untreated and future strokes are
not prevented, so many tiny strokes will occur that deep
and irreversible dementia will result. These may be severe

169

enough to irreparably impair vital memory. It is possible, however, to treat such patients and prevent future problems if the disease is found early enough. The following case is an illustration.

Alfred was the owner of a small dry-cleaning business who had a long history of heart disease with auricular fibrillation. When I saw him in one of the local Boston hospitals, he had an uneven gait and some loss of memory. In addition, other mental abilities were interfered with to the point that he could not run his business. A CAT scan taken in the course of his neurological evaluation showed tiny little strokes in the deep and superficial parts of his brain. This scan was made with one of the first CAT scanners to be set up in the northeastern United States, and the pictures were not as clear as those made by today's CAT scanners. But the diagnosis was unmistakable, and Alfred was put on blood thinners at age fifty-five.

I followed Alfred's case for twelve years. He recovered some of his mental powers, had no progression of his disease, and was able to function quite adequately with his wife in the dry-cleaning business until they sold it and retired to Florida.

The lesson is that the clinical picture of anyone with memory loss and other kinds of mental deterioration, along with loss of sensation or vision, weakness of an arm or a leg, or impaired coordination on one side, points to multi-infarct dementia rather than Alzheimer's disease, and the progression of this disorder can be arrested by anticoagulant treatment.

Finally, multi-infarct dementia, just like Alzheimer's, can be made much worse by depression, malnutrition, or brain poisoning with various sedative or psychiatric drugs as well as alcohol and street drugs like cocaine. Cocaine itself can produce tiny or large strokes even in young people who have no history of arterial disease or prior heart problems.

Multi-Infarct Dementia (Type II): Border Zone Infarct

In what is known as Binswanger's disease, or border zone infarct, another kind of tiny stroke occurs in the border zones of the brain when there isn't enough blood pressure to force the arterial blood through partially obstructed arteries. Persons taking an excess amount of antihypertensive medication can be susceptible to these strokes, particularly when they stand up and become hypotensive — that is, their blood pressure drops below normal levels.

If the periods of low blood pressure are long enough, tiny strokes occur in the inside part of the brain. The areas in which these strokes occur are the so-called watershed or border zones, which derive their name from the fact that they are located in the deep areas of the brain at the border between the part of the brain supplied by one artery (for example, the anterior cerebral artery) and a part of the brain supplied by another (the middle cerebral artery). The border zones are only marginally supplied by both arteries, and when a decrease in blood pressure results in decreased irrigation of blood through the brain, they may not get enough blood, producing a small stroke, or infarct. Disease of the small vessels of the brain, the penetrating blood vessels, is also often present.

Many doctors do not distinguish between the tiny strokes that occur in the border zones of the brain in Binswanger's disease and those that produce multi-infarct dementia type I, although I believe the two are quite separate entities. Taken together, these two stroke-producing conditions are frequent causes of lost intellectual function and memory loss. This is not only true in nursing home patients but also in people living independently at home. It's therefore essential that anyone whose intellectual or memory abilities have declined seek competent medical attention promptly and have a thorough evaluation to rule out these disorders, since these are problems that can be treated and prevented.

Blood Pressure: High and Low

One factor that has led to a great reduction in the incidence of strokes has been doctors' recognition that people with uncontrolled high blood pressure are much more likely to suffer strokes than people with normal blood pressure. Because of the beneficial effects of keeping blood pressure within normal limits, many doctors prescribe antihypertensive agents if patients have one or two blood pressure readings above accepted normal limits. They seem to think it is better to err on the side of keeping the blood pressure low than to take a chance on future stroke.

But high blood pressure is not the only factor that contributes to strokes. The same dietary problems that are related to premature heart attacks, namely, diets too high in saturated fats, may also be related to disease of the blood vessels in the brain and subsequent strokes. Even if a stroke does not occur, the narrowing of a blood vessel may make it more susceptible to low blood pressure. There just isn't enough pressure in the arterial blood vessels to force the blood through the narrowed, diseased arteries for a normal irrigation of brain tissue. This problem is more common with the widespread use of antihypertensive agents, even in people under age fifty.

Greg was a forty-three-year-old accountant whose high-stress existence, especially around tax time, kept him in a state of continual anxiety. Because his blood pressure was high, his doctor put him on antihypertensive medication. The problem with Greg was that he thought that if one antihypertensive pill was good for him, two were twice as good — so when he felt under stress, he doubled up on his medication.

Because Greg didn't recognize what was happening to himself, he inadvertently forced his blood pressure down below normal limits. He didn't pay attention to the warning signs —

particularly when he got up out of bed and felt dizzy and unsteady, as if he was going to topple over.

Greg took enough medication during tax time that he started to have lower-than-normal blood pressure even when he wasn't standing up, and he began to notice that he was unsteady when he walked. Worst of all, he began having difficulty with recent memory, and he appeared slowed down, depressed, and apathetic.

As an accomplished professional, Greg had always prided himself on his good memory, and a good memory was necessary to assist the diverse clients who used his services, each with their own individual and sometimes complicated problems. When he consulted me he was afraid he was getting Alzheimer's disease. But what I saw when I took a CAT scan of his brain tissue revealed quite a different picture. Because of his self-induced low blood pressure, he had had tiny little strokes in the border zones around the outer surface of the fluid-filled spaces of his brain.

I put Greg on an antidepressant medicine called Desyrel and referred him back to his internist for better control of his antihypertensive medication. Both his walking and his memory improved dramatically, even though the small strokes seen on his CAT scan stayed the same. The reason an antidepressant like Desyrel works in cases like Greg's is that border zone strokes destroy brain fibers that carry neurotransmitters. The antidepressant stimulant helps make up for the neurotransmitter deficiency.

Binswanger's disease, microvascular infarctions in the border zones of the brain leading to loss of intellectual capacity, is usually seen in people much older than Greg. Because CAT scans of older patients sometimes show a decrease in the density of border zone tissues not accompanied by specific mental changes, some doctors think the diagnosis of Binswanger's disease is overused. I disagree. In fact my partner, Tom Sabin, and his associate Gopal Venna have evidence that this syndrome, which is often made worse by antihypertensive drugs, is much more common than is generally recognized.

Controlling Your Own Blood Pressure

My point is to alert you to the fact that blood pressure should be neither too high nor too low. In no way do I mean to keep you from taking necessary medication to reduce high blood pressure, but it should be reserved for those who really need it. Some persons with mildly elevated blood pressure can be managed by diet alone — a diet not only low in fat but especially in saturated fat, and which also severely restricts salt (primarily sodium) intake.

Many of the foods you buy in the supermarket list the amount of sodium they contain on the labels. Read these labels. Going on a low-sodium diet requires more than just not putting added salt from a salt shaker on your food; it means avoiding many kinds of canned foods and soups that are simply loaded with sodium.

It's difficult to understand food producers who present items for sale which contain low amounts of salt but high amounts of saturated fats in the form of hydrogenated oil. Why would anyone who has to restrict intake of sodium want to buy low-salt peanut butter made with hydrogenated peanut oil? It doesn't make any sense nutritionally, and the manufacturers of such products should be educated to serve the best interests of the public by reducing not only sodium but also saturated and total fats in their products.

Another thing to remember about blood pressure level is that it may vary considerably depending on the level of exertion as well as the emotional state of the person being monitored. Some people get so anxious about the possibility of having high blood pressure that they actually send their blood pressure up when they are having it taken by a nurse or physician. It's important, obviously, to obtain a base-line reading for each patient. The art of getting a true reading, not a stressed one, may require considerable patience on the part of the medical care-giver.

Gwen, an amateur musician, had had rheumatic heart disease when she was sixteen which produced a loud murmur. She always dreaded going to the doctor because she was afraid her heart was defective, and that the defect would be obvious to any physician who listened to her chest. Her usual doctor retired when she was fifty-two and the new doctor who saw her was rather stiff and formal. Gwen became frightened when he took her blood pressure. It was 160. He had her come in again a week later, when it was even higher. It finally stabilized at 180; that's when he put her on antihypertensive medication, and one of the pills he gave her was the beta blocker propranolol. He also had her restrict her salt intake.

Gwen took the medication for six or seven months. During that time she felt more and more depressed and confused, and she was worried about her failing memory. Exasperated about her ill health, and without even asking her doctor, she stopped taking the medication but continued to restrict her salt intake. In a short time she felt much better and was much more alert, and her memory returned to normal.

Thirty years later, after she had moved to another state, Gwen broke her hip. She had her blood pressure taken a number of times, both before and after her hip replacement surgery and of course during the surgical procedure. Her blood pressure was absolutely normal, and it continued in the normal range until she died at the age of eighty-six.

The example of Gwen shows that if mild high blood pressure is treated in time (and if there is no kidney disease or diabetes), a low-salt diet may be adequate to prevent strokes. And, of course, blood pressure is unlikely to be too low when it is managed by diet alone.

Major Strokes and Memory Loss

In the popular mind, someone who has suffered a stroke becomes paralyzed on one side of the body, often with partial or total loss of speech. Indeed, many strokes present in just this way, but some instead result in a loss of a visual field, or of sensation in one part or one half of the body, as well as of intellectual and memory functions. Also, major strokes are sometimes correlated with major heart attacks, and it is not unusual for these two clinical problems to occur within six months of one another.

The factors that predispose a person to major stroke and heart attack are very similar. A genetic factor influences the way the body handles saturated fats and cholesterol, high blood pressure, and a high salt (sodium chloride) intake. Also, a diet rich in saturated fats, including such foods as pork, bacon, ham, tenderloin steaks, and often the tastiest cuts of meat (the taste is often in the saturated fat) as well as excessive amounts of butter, cream, ice cream, and whole milk (as opposed to skim milk), contributes to one's propensity for having either stroke or heart attack.

The list of foods high in saturated fats extends to hot dogs and hamburgers, some kinds of cheese, egg yolks, and many rich desserts such as cakes and pies made with vegetable shortening, lard, or hydrogenated oil. Combine this kind of diet with insufficient exercise, add some canned foods with high salt content, which increases the tendency toward high blood pressure, and just for good measure keep on smoking cigarettes, and you have a prescription for early heart attack and stroke, especially if your genetic makeup makes you predisposed to have such problems.

Memory loss can be the direct result of a stroke that involves the memory pathways, and particularly the inner parts of the temporal lobe. Millie, a seventy-six-year-old homemaker, had a single large stroke in one temporal lobe at age sixty-eight, and then some years later a second stroke in

176

the opposite temporal lobe after surgery to remove one of her breasts. Her second stroke left her with the physical symptom of only mild weakness, but it devastated her mentally: she suffered a completely incapacitating loss of recent memory. In effect, her vital memory was irreversibly destroyed, and she existed in a kind of time warp, unable to remember any of her ongoing experiences. Her children were disturbed by her symptoms and thought she had become insane. It was not of much comfort to Millie, but we were able to show her bewildered relatives the CAT scans of her two strokes. They understood the origin of her disabling symptoms and were able to provide her with sympathetic and appropriate supportive treatment.

Things to Be Aware Of

Memory loss occurs in people who have had strokes for several independent reasons. The first is the death of brain tissue (infarction) containing portions of the memory pathways. Secondary effects of the stroke such as depression, brain intoxication with prescription drugs, or malnutrition stemming from incapacity may also cause memory loss.

Finally, a possible cause of memory loss related to stroke is epileptic seizure. Such a seizure may occur early, at the time of the initial insult to the brain, or later, as the infarct scars over and begins to irritate surrounding brain tissue, resulting in a convulsion. In some patients these epileptic seizures are obvious, whereas in others very localized seizures can be easily missed, even by a trained observer. The seizures can affect the functioning of the memory pathways, producing transient amnesia, and if they are repeated the amnesia can be quite prolonged. The problem is treatable by antiseizure medication.

The best treatment for stroke is prevention through watching the diet, exercising, maintaining normal blood pressure, and avoiding tobacco, alcohol, and other drugs like cocaine which can produce strokes. When a stroke has occurred, however, it is important to examine the stroke victim carefully to see if memory has been affected. Preservation of memory, and especially vital memory, can be an essential stepping stone for rehabilitating movement, speech, and even certain aspects of intelligence.

In the rehabilitation process it is also necessary to keep the attention of stroke patients focused on something or someone besides themselves. Directing attention to an outside problem is the best way to avert depression. Secondary depression in someone who has suffered a stroke can be almost as disabling, as far as impairing memory is concerned, as the stroke itself, and its reversal can help preserve vital memory.

A patient who has had a stroke should have a CAT or MRI scan done, which will define the precise part of brain tissue which has been lost and assess the structure of the remaining brain tissue in the area of the stroke. Such an assessment can give a picture of the parts of the brain which are still structurally sound and capable of taking over lost brain function with the aid of directed rehabilitation therapy.

Finally even after restricting saturated fats and salt in your diet — and giving up smoking — you may require antihypertensive medicine prescribed by your physician. You should know, however, that not all of these medicines are equally safe or effective. Some antihypertensive drugs, called alpha blockers, not only lower blood pressure but also reduce the "bad" kinds of cholesterol in your blood. Get as much information about the medicine you'll be taking before you start your treatment, and be aware of both the potential benefits and the side effects.

Vital Memory Points to Remember

1. Multi-infarct dementia, which causes memory loss, is the result of tiny strokes that occur deep inside the brain.

2. Doctors sometimes confuse multi-infarct dementia with Alzheimer's disease.
3. Multi-infarct dementia is the second most common irreversible cause of memory loss and mental impairment.
4. Measures to prevent strokes include
   —following a low-fat diet (especially one restricted in saturated fats)
   —treating high blood pressure and avoiding low blood pressure
   —avoiding nicotine and tobacco
   —exercising moderately but regularly
   —avoiding excessive salt in the diet

17

Surgically Treatable Causes of Memory Loss

Subdural Hematomas

ANY OF US CAN get hit on the head hard enough to cause a blood clot pressing on the brain which may produce memory problems. Blood clots that press on the brain, most frequently the variety known as subdural hematomas, are called the "great imitators" because the signs and symptoms they produce can imitate many neurological and psychiatric syndromes. If the blood clots are toward the front of the brain, they can produce apathy and attention deficits. If they are farther back, they can produce weakness or numbness. And if they grow to large size, they can produce all these symptoms. Moreover, because they shift the brain stem, they can cause decreased consciousness, paralysis, and a change in pupil size.

These blood clots are also classified as to whether they occur acutely and produce dramatic changes in the brain or whether, as frequently happens, they expand slowly over a period of days or weeks. They are then often accompanied by headaches and a rather unusual tenderness and sensitivity of the scalp. Even the chronic ones, if left unattended over six to eight weeks, can produce a major loss of intellectual function, including a loss of memory abilities.

180

Chronic Subdural Hematomas in the Elderly

Chronic subdural hematomas are more frequent in the elderly than in people in their twenties and thirties. This diagnosis is often missed in patients who are unsteady and especially prone to fall and hit their heads. Many patients who have chronic subdural hematomas don't even recall that they've had a previous head injury, so a diagnosis is made on other grounds.

Connie was a seventy-six-year-old retired travel agent. She had had several small strokes, but her condition had stabilized and she was able to walk around and largely take care of herself. About six months before I saw her she had been admitted to another hospital where evaluation of her brain function, including a CAT scan of her brain, had been made without showing any remarkable deviations from normal.

One morning Connie seemed to grow faint in the shower and was a little dizzy. Her daughter thought she might have suffered another small stroke and also noted that her mother's memory wasn't as good as it had been before this episode, and that her walking was not as facile. Her daughter called the doctor, who told her to get Connie back to the hospital for a workup. But because Connie had had a normal CAT scan six months before, the emergency room doctor felt that it was unnecessary to repeat the examination, and he sent her home again.

Over the next three or four days, Connie had a bit more difficulty walking. A psychiatrist who saw her said that her trouble in walking, what he called the "leaning tower of Pisa syndrome," was not unusual in persons taking the tranquilizer she was on.

Her daughter, however, was not satisfied with this answer. She called the attending doctor and again asked him to have another examination done. Since the original hospital refused to do further examinations she brought Connie to my office, where we found that she had some weakness, especially in one leg (accounting for the "leaning tower" when she walked) and a loss of recent memory. A CAT scan of the brain showed an enormous blood clot pressing the brain from one side to the other. The clot was subsequently removed, with a fair return of memory and other intellectual functions.

It was a good thing Connie's daughter was so persistent. The blood clot had displaced brain tissue to the extent that Connie's life would have been in danger, or at least irreversible brain damage threatened, if diagnosis and treatment had been further delayed.

Occasionally small subdural hematomas will clear up without surgical drainage — but don't bank on it. Some patients treated conservatively by neurological physicians have succumbed to sudden shifts in pressure within their skulls. Except with very small hematomas, I believe that surgical evacuation is the wisest course in almost every case.

Ruling Out Subdural Hematomas as a Cause of Memory Loss

In any case of memory loss one should consider subdural hematoma as a possible cause that must be ruled out with a CAT scan or magnetic resonance imaging of the brain. This was especially true in the case of Elmer, a forty-nine-year-old shoe salesman admitted with a primary diagnosis of depression and memory loss to a nearby mental hospital. He was lucky that an astute neurologist was asked to consult on his case. Before allowing Elmer's psychiatrist to go further with medications or electroshock treatment, the neurologist asked for a CAT scan, which showed a large subdural hematoma that had produced a dangerous shift in brain structures.

The treatment of this man's problem by removing the hematoma was so gratifying, and the reversal of symptoms so prompt, that everyone was pleased — the psychiatrist, for discharging his patient as cured; the neurologist, for discovering the problem; but most of all the patient, who regained memory and mental functions after being misdiagnosed as having a severe, intractable depression.

Subdural hematoma is a great imitator of brain disability and disease, and even many psychiatric syndromes. In psychiatric and neurological cases in which the diagnosis is in doubt, a CAT or MRI scan is simple to do and will rule out this completely treatable problem.

Brain Tumors

What would you think if your doctor told you that the cause of your memory loss was a brain tumor? First and foremost, you need not panic. Many brain tumors are benign, and with modern surgical techniques they can be cured. Second, don't imagine that your doctor is likely to find that your symptoms are caused by a brain tumor. Unlike what you may have been led to believe by watching television soap operas or reading sensational tabloids, brain tumors are relatively uncommon in our population, constituting about 2 percent of all the tumors found in humans.

What you must keep in mind is that most brain tumors are treatable and many are curable, together with their symptom of memory loss if it occurs. Brain tumors must be diagnosed early, however; if left untreated, the increased pressure within the head which they generate will impair not only memory but many other brain functions. They interfere with normal brain function either by just the mass effect of the tumor itself, or by obstructing the flow of spinal fluid, causing a backup and expansion of the fluid spaces in the brain in the condition called hydrocephalus. The increased pressure is relayed into the backs of the eyeballs, where the optic nerve heads are located, and these structures tend to swell, causing a loss of vision.

Brain tumors, of course, damage brain tissue locally by direct pressure on the tissue, and there is often additional damage to the surrounding brain because of swelling or edema caused by the advancing tumor itself. A tumor can also interfere with the blood supply to the brain, and, of course, it can irritate the brain tissue around it to produce epileptic seizures.

How Brain Tumors Affect Memory

Even when a brain tumor doesn't invade memory pathways, it may still impede mental processes and recent memory because of increased pressure and its effects within the head. That's what happened to Andy, a fifty-two-year-old carpet cleansing manager, before he entered the hospital. About nine months prior to when I saw him he had complained to his physicians of severe pain in his head, which was worse when he put his head forward or changed its position suddenly. Shortly afterward his business associates noted that he was not as sharp in his business dealings or as responsible as he had been. The company he worked for started to lose money because of the decisions Andy made, and in a desperate effort to recoup some of it for them, Andy made choices that only made matters worse.

When I saw him, Andy walked with a wide-based gait and was unsteady on his feet. His optic nerve heads were swollen, indicating that he had increased pressure in his brain, and he had a major loss of intellectual function and particular difficulty with recent memory.

Special x-ray tests showed that he had a tumor in the back part of his brain which obstructed the flow of spinal fluid, producing hydrocephalus. Subsequently the mass was completely removed by surgery, and he had a dramatic recovery. The increased pressure in his head subsided completely and his intellectual ability returned, with vast improvement of his recent memory. Unfortunately, the return of his mental abilities didn't happen in time to save his job. With his previous contacts and his regained health, however, he found new

employment and now has a good chance to become successful again in the commercial marketplace.

Other Types of Brain Tumors That Affect Memory

The type of tumor Andy had, a glioma, is the most common
variety. Other kinds can bring about similar but different
symptoms. A slow-growing tumor in the front part of the
brain (a meningioma) can produce gradual deterioration in
intellectual abilities and memory which may escape notice for
a number of years. That was the situation in the case of Helga,
a forty-seven-year-old business executive who owned an ex-
clusive and profitable modeling agency and who also manufactured and distributed cosmetics. I was asked to see her
after she had been charged by the Internal Revenue Service
with evading $2.3 million in taxes over a three-year period.

Her defense at first didn't seem very good. She claimed not
to have any memory of conferences with her lawyers or with
IRS agents, conferences that were critical to the case against
her. Helga was unlike the typical person charged with tax
evasion, however. Well after the IRS investigation of her finances started, she began to have difficulty with her vision,
and it was noticed that her optic nerve head was swollen and
she had increased pressure in her brain. CAT scans and magnetic resonance images showed a slow-growing tumor in the
front part of her brain which was as big as a tangerine. It
threatened her life and was promptly removed. But even after
surgery her personality did not revert to normal, although
her brain function, including recent memory, gradually improved.

The tumor had not only compressed part of her brain but
also obstructed its blood supply. The resultant scarring in the
area generated occasional epileptic seizures. Because the tumor had been in the frontal rather than the temporal lobes, it
didn't directly interfere with the memory circuits. It did, however, through interrupting frontal lobe function, produce ap-

athy, a symptom hard to distinguish from severe depression in its effects on concentration and attention. Thus the tumor disturbed the acquisition of new memories, and it slowed Helga's ability to retrieve memories from her memory bank.

The removal of Helga's brain tumor improved her memory abilities, but they were still intermittently and unpredictably disrupted by the localized epileptic seizures at the site where the brain tumor had been. Subsequently her memory was further improved by the administration of antiseizure drugs. As for her troubles with the IRS, the government has a rather weak case against her, and I think she will ultimately win. No one with a sizable tumor like Helga's should be convicted of tax evasion.

Once a tumor is suspected, diagnosis can be readily made with imaging techniques like CAT and MRI scans. Making such a diagnosis early is crucial because early treatment, whether by surgical excision or sometimes radiation therapy, not only improves the chances that a complete cure will be effected but can also relieve symptoms and reverse memory loss.

Hydrocephalus

Guess what Beethoven and Amenhotep IV, the pharaoh who introduced the worship of a single God in Egypt, had in common. All right, you give up? Both suffered the condition known as arrested hydrocephalus, a clinical problem that, in its controlled state, is compatible with great mental ability. Progressive hydrocephalus, however, whether caused by an obstruction such as a brain tumor or a constriction of the outflow ducts, will produce increased pressure within the skull and a significant decrease in intellectual and memory functions.

Elderly people tend to get a kind of hydrocephalus or accumulation of excess spinal fluid, with dilatation of the

186

fluid-filled spaces, or ventricles, in the brain, without having increased pressure inside the head. This condition, called normal-pressure hydrocephalus, results from lowered brain elasticity, which allows any temporary increase in pressure in the ventricles to balloon them out. The effects on brain function — including loss of memory, incontinence, and especially difficulty walking — are great, even though the pressure inside the head remains normal.

To illustrate, I'd like to relate the case of Martha, seventy-two, who was a hard-working short-order cook and waitress who had successively helped support two alcoholic husbands, whom she divorced, and another who died of a heart attack. Martha had a long history of manic-depressive disease and was hospitalized on several occasions for many months. When I saw her she complained of "wicked" headaches and had severe difficulty walking. In fact, she couldn't walk without the aid of a three-pronged cane, and even then she seemed to stagger from one side of the hall to the other. The nurse who accompanied her said that, in addition, her memory was gone; she couldn't remember anything. "She lives from one minute to the next. I have to dress her and feed her," the nurse said.

A CAT scan of Martha's brain showed hugely dilated ventricles, way out of proportion to the shrinkage in the rest of her brain. Now hydrocephalus can be treated by an operation that shunts the spinal fluid through a one-way valve into the abdominal cavity, or even into the heart. But first radioactive tests need to be done to trace the flow of spinal fluid and confirm the diagnosis. I find one of the more reliable predictive indicators of successful surgical treatment to be repeated spinal punctures, with the removal of spinal fluid. If the removal of spinal fluid improves memory and especially walking, the shunting procedure has a high chance of being effective. Because preliminary removal of spinal fluid gave her temporary relief from her symptoms on several occasions, Martha is scheduled for surgery in the near future, and I have high hopes that it will be successful.

The shunting procedure in older patients with hydrocephalus has lost popularity among some physicians because dementia and memory loss are not reversed in a few patients. This result is not because the operation doesn't remove the excess spinal fluid; it is rather that these patients actually have two diseases: hydrocephalus and Alzheimer's disease or Binswanger's disease (border zone infarcts), which also allows the ventricles to dilate. Of course, surgical treatment is not effective for either of the latter conditions. Even in Alzheimer's patients with hydrocephalus, however, improvement in walking is often noted.

Hydrocephalus can be ruled out with a CAT scan or magnetic resonance imaging, and thus it will be picked up on the usual battery of tests given to patients who have memory loss or other deterioration in their mental abilities. It is good to keep in mind that hydrocephalus can also be a consequence of brain injury or brain hemorrhage, and that mental deterioration or persistent memory loss in patients demands proper imaging of the brain to rule out this treatable and reversible problem.

Hydrocephalus and Aggressive Behavior

Kenneth, an eighty-two-year-old candy store owner, was a kindly widower who spent much of his time serving the young customers who came to his shop on their way home from school. One spring afternoon a child who had visited his store stepped off the sidewalk in front of a car, and Kenneth rushed into the street, pushed the child out of the way, and was himself hit by the motorist, who had vainly tried to stop. Kenneth was unconscious for a while and was sent to a neighborhood hospital, where he was found to have blood in his spinal fluid. He recovered over a period of four or five days, and after a ten-day period he was sent to stay with his son and daughter-in-law.

Kenneth's behavior became more unusual as the weeks passed. Unlike most hydrocephalic patients, who become sleepy and lethargic, Kenneth became quite aggressive. He also had memory loss and occasional incontinence. One morning while he was shaving himself with a straight razor he whipped it around and threatened his daughter-in-law, saying, "I'm going to cut your head off." She ran screaming from the apartment.

When Kenneth was brought into the hospital he had very pronounced hydrocephalus, which was treated by the shunting procedure. When he awoke from surgery he told the female resident who was taking care of him, "Kiss me, sweetie, or I'll punch you in the nose." Over the next several days, however, he improved remarkably, and his aggressive tendencies disappeared. Kenneth's memory also improved, and his walking was quite stable.

Proper Diagnosis

Cases like Kenneth's are unusual because, as noted above, most people with this disorder experience lethargy along with other symptoms such as recent-memory loss, trouble walking and a tendency to fall, and incontinence. The lesson to remember as far as hydrocephalus is concerned is the same one conveyed in the previous sections on subdural hematomas and brain tumors: when the diagnosis is in doubt, include a CAT scan or magnetic resonance imaging in the patient's evaluation. These techniques allow us not only to diagnose but to visualize in detail well over 90 percent of all the surgically treatable problems of the brain discussed in this chapter. I also feel strongly that the use of these diagnostic tools should be considered for persons with unexplained psychiatric symptoms, including personality changes, as well as for patients with obvious brain disease.

Vital Memory Points to Remember

1. Subdural hematomas are blood clots that press on the brain whose effects can imitate many different neurological and psychiatric syndromes.
2. Brain tumors often interfere with mental processes and recent memory because of increased pressure within the head.
3. Prompt diagnosis of these problems by CAT scan or magnetic resonance imaging allows early treatment to be undertaken and therefore improves outcomes.

18

Degenerative Brain Disease and Memory Loss

THE DEGENERATIVE BRAIN DISORDERS are those characterized by a loss of brain tissue and corresponding mental function. Some of these disorders, such as multiple sclerosis, have a sputtering course; they flare up for a while, then a period of months or even years may ensue in which there are no symptoms. Others, like Parkinson's disease, progress slowly but steadily, causing a loss of tissue and a deficiency of neurotransmitters deep in the brain. Still others, like Alzheimer's, have a more rapid course, producing a loss of tissue in the cortex, the surface of the brain.

In this chapter I concentrate on Alzheimer's because it is the most frequent cause of irreversible memory loss in the elderly. The onset of this disease may vary, but memory problems — particularly loss of recent memory — is always prominent. Some people with the disease have degeneration in the speech areas of the brain, making it difficult for them to name objects. Tissue degeneration in others disturbs their orientation — for example, their ability to find their destination in a car or even on foot. Whatever the pattern of brain loss, it progresses until all of the above symptoms of brain loss are prominent. The patterns themselves are not invariable, however, and it is likely that the name Alzheimer's describes more than one degenerative brain disease.

The words *Alzheimer's disease* are among the most feared in the vocabularies of persons over the age of forty-five because they raise the specter of irreversible and devastating memory loss and mental helplessness. People seem to feel that there is a certain inevitability about the disease, and many (including some doctors) equate it with aging or senility.

Myths About Alzheimer's Disease

To begin this discussion of Alzheimer's disease, I'd like to dispel some myths about it. First, normal aging does not produce senility or Alzheimer's. That is a well-established medical fact. Second, although Alzheimer's is a diagnosis of exclusion, only to be confirmed by the characteristic changes in the brain seen at post-mortem examination, its clinical picture may represent more than one disease with different causes and, eventually, quite different treatments. Third, although some people have a genetic predisposition to develop Alzheimer's disease, which is perhaps more strongly manifested in victims who get the disorder before the age of fifty-five, inheritance doesn't explain all the factors that lead to the clinical expression of the disease.

Causes of Alzheimer's Disease

There are lots of theories about what causes Alzheimer's. Early in 1991, Dr. John Hardy of St. Mary's Hospital in London announced that he and his colleagues had discovered at least one of the genes that cause Alzheimer's. According to the researchers, a mutation occurs in the gene which directs cells to produce a protein called beta amyloid, a component of nerve cells. It is this protein that is thought to be responsible for the disease. Dr. Hardy's research appears to be quite promising and may yet reveal both a cause and a cure for Alzheimer's.

192

Slow viral infections of the brain have been raised as a possible inciting factor. Also, the ingestion of certain metals, such as aluminum, has been under investigation (I must add without much in the way of convincing evidence). Decreased lecithin or choline has been put forward as a cause of the loss of cells in the cholinergic circuit related to the memory process. The overaccumulation of organic compounds related to glutamate (glutamic acid), which kills nerve cells by producing an excess amount of calcium around them, has been suggested as a mechanism in various degenerative brain diseases. Other proposed factors include chronic alcohol abuse with repeated head injury and even poor intellectual attainment.

Diagnosis of Alzheimer's Disease

Researchers in a number of centers are working on ways to enable us to make a positive diagnosis of Alzheimer's disease before death. One of the more promising leads is the discovery of a protein in the brain which is present in about 85 percent of people who have the diagnosis of Alzheimer's confirmed at post-mortem examination. This substance may be present in the spinal fluid as well, and thus a positive diagnosis might be possible by identifying this protein in specimens of spinal fluid obtained by lumbar puncture.

I personally believe that it is a mistake to concentrate on early diagnosis of Alzheimer's disease before there is effective treatment. Once the diagnosis of Alzheimer's disease is established, too many physicians give up any attempt to search out other treatable problems that might be making the Alzheimer's patient worse, and the patient is prematurely sent to a nursing home. Tests should therefore be used only in the end stages of the disease, and in the meantime we should continue to look for conditions (even in suspected Alzheimer's cases) that are treatable and reversible. The role of the much-publicized abnormal protein in Alzheimer's should

193

not be underestimated, however, since it may well be the key to determining the causal mechanisms in many cases of the disease, and in turn to discovering effective treatment and prevention strategies.

Radioactive PET and Spect (single photon emission computerized tomography) scans detect abnormally reduced metabolism in certain areas of the brain in Alzheimer's patients. But caution is necessary: other degenerative diseases that at post-mortem prove not to be Alzheimer's can have a similar radioactive scan pattern. Also, brain mapping using quantitative brain wave recordings shows slower activity in Alzheimer's patients than in depressed patients.

Dealing with Alzheimer's

Most patients with Alzheimer's disease don't complain about memory loss or their failing mental abilities because the critical faculty in the brain which allows them to monitor their own behavior is often lost quite early in the course of the illness. That is not to say that some patients with Alzheimer's are not quite depressed and fearful about what's happening to them, but this is usually not the case. Most people who come into my office with detailed complaints about their loss of memory are suffering from one of the reversible disorders, most commonly depression.

Another misconception about Alzheimer's is that it only occurs after the age of fifty. The frequency of its occurrence does increase after fifty, and even more after eighty, but it's a disorder that can occur at any age. Especially in children with Down's syndrome, Alzheimer's disease can manifest itself as early as age fifteen or sixteen.

I was recently challenged by an official at the National Institute of Aging when I said that even skillful neurologists are mistaken in their diagnosis of Alzheimer's disease in 12 to 20 percent of cases. My comment was based on the results of a study done at the University of Toronto's Sunnybrook Medical Center which reviewed post-mortem examinations of the brains of patients who, when they were alive, had been diagnosed by more than one doctor as having Alzheimer's disease. More than 14 percent of these patients had actually had a problem other than Alzheimer's.

The doctor who questioned my information said that recent studies using magnetic resonance imaging as well as new psychological research brought the error rate down to between 5 and 10 percent. Nevertheless, I maintain that he was overly optimistic and that the brains of many patients with the symptoms of Alzheimer's still do not, at post-mortem examinations, display the typical characteristics of the disease. In fact, some post-mortems have revealed the signs of Alzheimer's disease in patients who had had none of the symptoms. All this means is that there is a good deal of uncertainty about the diagnosis even among very experienced neurologists at major medical centers. If we were to consider the diagnosis of this disorder in general medical practice, we would have a much higher error rate, probably approaching 30 percent.

Reversible Complications in Alzheimer's Patients

The progression of Alzheimer's disease from slight to very severe dementia varies from individual to individual. Even when the disease is properly diagnosed, it can be still complicated by a number of other factors which make the symptoms much worse. Disorders like depression, brain poisoning with alcohol or prescription drugs, malnutrition, and even sensory monotony can nudge a patient who would be marginally self-sufficient into a state of complete dependence. That's why it's so important to check for treatable disorders even in patients who do have Alzheimer's. The correction of treatable problems can improve patients' clinical pictures enough so that they will be able to function independently for a much longer period of time than they would if

195

these problems were neglected. These additional causes of memory loss are more likely to occur in the nursing home setting, where sensory deprivation, depression, and especially brain poisoning with prescription drugs are all too common.

Degenerative Diseases Similar to Alzheimer's

Almost any degenerative brain disease may progress to the point that loss of memory and of intellectual function occurs, although mental impairment is much less common in the early stages of multiple sclerosis and Parkinson's disease. The time course varies greatly in the different disorders. Memory loss and mental deterioration are, of course, the hallmarks of Alzheimer's from the onset of the syndrome. By contrast, people with multiple sclerosis can remain static for decades, with no sign of mental deterioration or memory loss, whereas Parkinson's disease usually advances more quickly.

The fact that a disease is hereditary, as some cases of Alzheimer's may well be, does not mean that it is untreatable. Wilson's disease, for example, an inherited disorder causing degeneration of the inner parts of the brain and portions of the liver, may start as early as the second decade of life with a tremor of the limbs and head, slowness of movement, abnormal behavior, and finally loss of intellectual function, with loss of memory among other symptoms. Medical researchers have found that the genetic deficiency that causes Wilson's disease works by producing abnormally large deposits of copper, especially in the liver and brain. When these concentrations are reduced the symptoms of the disease can often be reversed, and many patients are brought back to normal brain function. Just as we have been able to treat the inherited brain defect that produces Wilson's disease, within the next ten to fifteen years we will be able to do the same for those patients who have inherited Alzheimer's disease.

One of the most difficult messages to deliver to families in which a member is stricken with an incurable degenerative brain disease is the message that they must not give up hope. Even if we don't now have an effective treatment for Alzheimer's disease, extensive research is being done which may lead to its eventual prevention and cure. And even when brain tissue has been lost, we may in the future be able to replace it with fetal nerve cell transplants.

In the meantime, and to reiterate my point on the treatment of patients with Alzheimer's disease, we must make every effort to diagnose other conditions that may make the symptoms of Alzheimer's, especially its attendant memory loss, worse than they need to be, and to treat those problems that are reversible promptly. Moreover, I want to stress to care-givers the importance of providing Alzheimer's victims every memory aid available. Such aids include establishing a firm and consistent routine to keep patients in one location, prominently displaying dates and times in large block letters near patients' beds or chairs, and making rooms they use easily accessible so that they can carry on their usual routines without getting lost. For example, ensure that they can get to the bathroom by themselves, and guard against their being able to lock themselves in or out. Also, doorways leading outside or to other potentially dangerous areas should be locked to prevent wandering in strange and difficult places.

Finally, care-givers to persons with Alzheimer's must learn to provide the level of assistance that is needed without smothering the abilities that patients still have for independent action. This means assessing their individual abilities and offering only the amount of help necessary for safety. It also means exercising patience in allowing patients to express their remaining talents, even if these are much reduced in quality, spontaneity, and speed. It means supporting them when they are frustrated and encouraging them when they falter. It means not getting angry when they make mistakes and never taking their anger or hostility seriously.

From this catalogue you can see how difficult it is to be a care-giver to an Alzheimer's patient. Imagine how much more difficult it would be for a member of the family to assume the role. Unlike a nurse who steps into the care-giving function from outside, family members can't forget how their loved one was before, and they can't stop mentally comparing the patient's present invalidism with past prowess.

It is gratifying, nevertheless, to hear the story of a man who was devotedly cared for by his sister, who kept him in the home he'd lived in for more than forty-five years. For fifteen years after he became ill with Alzheimer's disease, his sister guided him, with increasing assistance as time went on, in an unvarying routine, including seeing the same people at the same time each day. Even though he progressively lost brain tissue, he was able to live and function for a much longer period than most Alzheimer's victims.

Obviously, Alzheimer's disease varies in its intensity and rate of progression from person to person. We must therefore fit the treatment and the circumstances to each individual and not push patients prematurely into institutions that will make their intellectual and memory deficits worse. Let me emphasize that there *are* some people whose brain disease has advanced to such an extent that they are helpless. Unless they are well-to-do and can afford round-the-clock nursing care, institutionalization is the only alternative available to them. My plea is that institutionalization not occur until absolutely necessary. I have seen too many lives wasted that could otherwise have been productive in the so-called golden years, had complete diagnosis and correct treatment been carried out.

Vital Memory Points to Remember

1. Normal aging does not produce senility or Alzheimer's disease.
2. Alzheimer's, as a specific variety of dementia, is a diagnosis of exclusion which is usually only positively confirmed at post-mortem.
3. Genetics does not explain all the factors that lead to Alzheimer's. Do not think that just because one of your parents has Alzheimer's you are destined to get it.
4. A diagnosis of Alzheimer's disease does not necessarily mean that the patient is incompetent. I have seen Alzheimer's patients who, while disabled in one sphere, were competent in another — finance, say, or ornamental gardening. The degree of incompetence depends on the extent of tissue loss in the cortex of the brain in each patient.
5. Treatable causes of dementia may be present in Alzheimer's patients, and these conditions may make memory loss much worse than it needs to be. These disorders should be diagnosed and treated promptly.
6. Memory aids, a predictable routine, and intelligent patient monitoring are the essence of effective management of Alzheimer's patients. Patients should be given enough independence to express their abilities and enough supervision to compensate for their deficits. The level of freedom has to be determined for each individual.
7. Advances in diagnostic methods offer hope that not only successful treatments for the symptoms of Alzheimer's but also techniques for preventing its progression will be developed.

Hope for the Future

19

Prevention: What You Can Do to Avoid Memory Loss

OVER THE LAST YEAR I've traveled through much of the eastern part of the United States, and I've had the chance to be on radio talk shows broadcast to the whole nation. The questions and concerns voiced from Alaska, California, and Oklahoma are much the same as those from New York, Pennsylvania, and Florida. Everyone wants to know what can be done to prevent a decline in memory and other intellectual functions and prolong useful life. I would like to review with you some of the questions I've been asked about memory loss and what treatments might reverse it, as well as about preventing memory loss and intellectual deterioration.

Preventing Memory Loss Associated with Alzheimer's

The question I hear most often is, "How can I prevent memory loss and keep from getting Alzheimer's disease?" At the present time we don't know precisely what causes Alzheimer's disease, and this knowledge is necessary for prevention. We think there may be an inherited predisposition in some cases, probably a minority of the cases. And this predisposition is more pronounced in persons who are afflicted with the disease before the age of fifty-five.

Statistical studies reviewed and reported by A. S. Henderson, a researcher in social psychiatry from the Australian National University in Canberra, report that the number of people showing clinical signs and symptoms of Alzheimer's disease increases consistently with age. He concluded that the process underlying the dementia that characterizes Alzheimer's becomes more intense with age. The peculiar thing about these statistics, however, is that the increase in the incidence of Alzheimer's disease with age stops abruptly at age ninety, when it begins to go down. We thus know that aging in itself is not a cause of the disease.

It has also been reported that more women than men have Alzheimer's, and that more men than women have multi-infarct dementia (small strokes). However, this observation may be biased because, since women live longer than men, there are more women in the older age groups that have a greater incidence of Alzheimer's disease.

It's also interesting to note that studies have been undertaken to differentiate the vulnerability of individuals to Alzheimer's disease on the basis of their social class and education. Several studies found the incidence of Alzheimer's disease among the well educated to be thirty times less than it is among the poorly educated. Because they are controversial, studies such as these have been criticized as being biased. In my opinion, the results are certainly astonishing, and there is no biological explanation for them. Furthermore, they don't square with my own experience, which is that well-to-do, highly educated people appear to get Alzheimer's disease as often as anyone else.

Correlates with Alzheimer's disease are a history of blood transfusion, a previous diagnosis of clinical depression, and a history of herpes zoster, a viral disease commonly known as shingles. Some researchers investigating the disease have also noted an association between the primary dementia, or loss of intellectual function, and a past history of diabetes, physical inactivity, heart disease (particularly heart failure), and constipation. Alzheimer's disease and multi-infarct dementia occur together much more often than just by chance. It may be that the multiple small cerebral infarcts accelerate the clinical course — that is, increase the loss of memory and other intellectual functions which occurs in Alzheimer's.

Head injuries too have been implicated as a co-factor with Alzheimer's disease in two studies that found some statistical correlations between the two phenomena. Six other studies have failed to find the correlation, however, and in two others the correlation was not significant.

The question has been raised as to whether any medications have been linked to Alzheimer's disease, and indeed studies have linked the pain reliever Phenacitin to changes in the brain which resemble the characteristics of Alzheimer's disease.

What risk factors are associated with Alzheimer's? Dr. J. Mortimer of the University of Minnesota has suggested that a family history of dementia is the most frequent risk factor, and prior head trauma the second most common factor. Other risk factors that have been suggested, without much evidence, include the use of antiperspirants containing aluminum since increased levels of aluminum are among the pathological changes in the brains of Alzheimer's patients.

The possible role of aluminum in Alzheimer's disease has been widely publicized, causing a measure of hysteria in various communities in this country. In one case that I know about, the publicity caused an elderly woman to take drastic measures. Angelina, an eighty-six-year-old widow, was a meticulous housekeeper who collected bone china, dishes, and fine cooking utensils. Among other things, she had a collection of exquisite aluminum cookware and teapots. Angelina read somewhere about the theoretical connection between aluminum and Alzheimer's disease and how it afflicted people over the age of seventy-five. She immediately called her daughter to come over and dispose of every fine piece of aluminum in her collection.

What Angelina and many other people don't understand is that processes in the body reduce the amount of aluminum absorbed, particularly from the gastrointestinal tract. Also, many people don't realize that a number of commonly ingested antacids contain aluminum. Moreover, all of us take in a certain amount of aluminum in our food. If the metal did have a significant relationship with Alzheimer's disease, one would expect to see this disease cropping up in all those persons who have gastric disorders and are forced to take various antacid preparations. Since this is not the case, I believe that the relationship between aluminum ingestion and Alzheimer's disease is not substantiated.

What about alcohol consumption? Is there any link between use of alcohol and the onset of Alzheimer's? Indirect evidence exists about the connection between brain injury and Alzheimer's disease, and of course brain injury can in turn be caused by alcohol abuse. In addition, factors such as vitamin deficiencies and seizures stemming from alcoholism tend to confound the role of alcohol abuse in producing various syndromes that entail memory loss. There is evidence, however, that brain poisoning by alcohol can in itself reduce memory power. Alcohol-related dementia associated with atrophy of the brain and major loss of intellectual power, including vital memory, can also occur, though usually at a much younger age than Alzheimer's disease.

But although new discoveries have yielded tantalizing clues, I repeat that we don't yet know the exact cause of Alzheimer's disease and therefore have no sure method of prevention. This situation may well change in the next five years, but for now we can only hope that funding of basic research continues until a breakthrough comes.

Reducing Our Risk of Memory Loss

Brain Injury

We don't know enough yet to make specific recommendations for preventing Alzheimer's disease, but the risk factors for some other serious threats are only too well known.

Of utmost importance is the prevention of serious brain injury. Over half a million people in the United States suffer brain injuries related to automobile accidents each year; one hundred thousand of these injuries are serious. One of the most effective preventive measures is to have air bags fitted into every vehicle on the streets and highways of this country. Air bags, along with the use of three-point seat belt restraints, would markedly diminish the incidence of brain injuries. In addition, requiring appropriate helmets to be worn by players in all contact sports as well as by anyone riding a two- or three-wheel vehicle would be of great help.

And to take a public health approach to a grievous social problem, we should make every effort to lower the incidence of a mounting source of brain injury: gunshot wounds to the head. The streets of many American cities have become like war zones, with random shootings devastating the lives of not only those dealing in illegal drugs but also innocent bystanders. In the armed services, metal helmets are worn to reduce the velocity of bullets and shrapnel; instead of a high-velocity missile injury of the brain, a low-velocity missile wound results if the fragment penetrates the metal helmet, with consequent reduction in brain injury. What should we do in our urban areas? Issue infantry helmets to the residents — men, women, and children — of the inner city? Perhaps a more effective proposal would be to license persons who have guns of any sort inside the limits of our major urban areas, with severe penalties for anyone caught with an unlicensed gun.

Brain Poisoning

What role does brain poisoning play in premature loss of intellectual and memory functions? A very large one, in my view, among the more than six million alcoholics in this country as well as the millions who abuse cocaine, marijuana, Angel Dust, amphetamines, barbiturates, and other street drugs. Brain function is obviously impaired during the acute period of brain poisoning by alcohol or any of the street drugs, which cause a breakdown of the blood-brain barrier. This impairment can be as severe as that produced by a brain tumor, brain injury, or brain infection; the only difference is that brain function will return once the level of poisoning has abated. The chronic use of these brain poisons, however, is associated with the early onset of memory loss and deterioration of other intellectual powers. As I see it, the less these poisons are used, the better.

You should also try to minimize the use of various brain toxins that are medically prescribed, particularly the sedative hypnotics such as Ativan, Valium, Xanax, and Halcyon as well as the barbiturates, the bromides, and the major psychiatric drugs such as Stelazine, haloperidol, Thorazine, and lithium. In addition, drugs used in general medicine — digitalis, pain relievers, drugs used to control hypertension and diabetes, cimetidine, beta blockers (such as Inderal), Reserpine, Symmetrel, and drugs like Elavil that have anticholinergic actions (that is, are antagonistic to the neurotransmitter acetylcholine) — are potentially toxic to brain and memory function.

Obviously, you should not abandon medications prescribed by your doctor, even psychiatric medications, if they're clinically indicated. If you are losing memory or are having periods of confusion, however, you should go to your doctor and ask that the dosage be adjusted so you still get the therapeutic effect without the toxic or adverse reactions some of these drugs produce. Also, at times it's possible for your physician to substitute one drug for another to achieve the same therapeutic effect without the toxic side effect on the brain. Moreover, if you're taking a number of drugs for various medical problems, be sure your doctor knows about all the medications you're on, because sometimes combinations of drugs are more toxic to the brain than a single drug alone. Combinations of Mellaril and lithium or haloperidol and methyldopa, for example, are especially likely to produce loss of memory, confusion, and intellectual deterioration. Among the drugs reviewed should be eye drops for glaucoma and skin patches to prevent seasickness.

It is also important to avoid chemicals and pollutants in auto emissions and industrial waste products. Carbon dioxide, carbon monoxide, organic solvents, mercury, lead, and arsenic are simply a few of the many poisons that can contaminate our air, food chain, and water supply and adversely affect brain function and memory.

Diet and Memory Loss

Another frequently asked question about prevention is, "What about diet? Is what I eat important in keeping me mentally alert?" The answer is an unequivocal yes. Diet is crucial at all stages of the life cycle, especially during the prenatal period and in infancy, when the developing brain is extremely sensitive to nutritional deficiencies. Serial studies have shown that a lack of essential nutrients can affect certain neurotransmitter systems in the brain at the earliest stages of life, and the damage is never really fully corrected even when an adequate diet is initiated.

Many nutritionists will tell you that it's not necessary to take dietary supplements if your intake of cereals and grains, vegetables and fruits, milk products, and meat and fish is adequate. The unfortunate thing is that our lifestyles may preclude getting an adequate diet. Fast foods and processed foods may not contain the nourishment you need for your brain. Furthermore, as we get older we tend to be more sedentary and use fewer calories, so we eat less food, and the essential vitamins and nutrients may therefore be lacking in sufficient quantity. In addition, some people lose teeth as they grow older, and as a result they can't chew food properly and derive the full nutritional benefit from what they do eat.

I don't believe in megadoses of vitamins, but I also think that the optimal level of vitamins is greater than the classical nutritionists state. Therefore, I recommend the daily vitamin supplements listed in Table 2. These substances form the basis of adequate supplemental nutrition for the brain. Most of them are incorporated in a tablet that my partner, Tom Sabin, and I devised for the Schiff Company, a manufacturer of food supplements for health stores throughout the United States. In addition, I myself like to take a supplement of purified choline (phosphatidyl choline, or lecithin). I realize that some choline is manufactured in the body, and that the

TABLE 2 **Recommended Daily Minimum and Optimal Allowances of Vitamins and Minerals (For Adults and Children Ten Years Old and Older)[a]**

	Minimum	Optimal
Vitamins		
Vitamin A	5000 IU[b]	10,000 IU
Vitamin D	400 IU	400 IU
Vitamin E	30 IU	100 IU
Vitamin C	60.0 mg	1000.0 mg
Vitamin B_1 (thiamine)	1.5 mg	20.0 mg

TABLE 2 CONTINUED

	Minimum	Optimal
Vitamin B$_2$ (riboflavin)	1.7 mg	10.0 mg
Vitamin B$_3$ (niacin)	20.0 mg	250.0 mg
Vitamin B$_5$ (pantothenic acid)	10.0 mg	20.0 mg
Vitamin B$_6$ (pyridoxine)	2.0 mg	20.0 mg
Vitamin B$_9$ (folic acid)	400.0 mcg	400.0 mcg
Vitamin B$_{12}$ (cobalamines)	6.0 mcg	100.0 mcg
Vitamin H[c] (biotin)	n/a	300.0 mcg
Choline[d]	n/a	3.0 g
Minerals		
Calcium[e]	1.0 g	1.6 g
Phosphorus[e]	1.0 g	1.6 g
Iodine	150.0 mcg	150.0 mcg
Iron	18.0 mg	20.0 mg
Magnesium	400.0 mg	400.0 mg
Copper	2.0 mg	3.0 mg
Zinc	15.0 mg	25.0 mg
Other		
Spring water	n/a	1.5–2.0 liters (45–60 oz.)

[a]For persons who do not have allergies to specific foods containing these vitamins and for those who don't have diabetes or liver, thyroid, or kidney disease. Vitamin or nutritional supplements may be necessary for people who have allergies or intolerances to foods like milk, cheese, nuts, or fish. Nonallergenic food supplements are available and are strongly recommended to overcome the potential nutritional deficiencies that would otherwise occur in persons intolerant to basic foods.

[b]IU stands for international units, an international standard for measuring quantities of substances such as vitamins.

[c]Various amounts of this vitamin are normally produced in the intestine.

[d]Many nutritionists do not consider choline to be a vitamin because some amount of it is produced in the body, but I consider it so important that you may need to supplement it.

[e]You may substitute 3.2 grams per day of calcium phosphate.

statistical evidence that this substance enhances memory is equivocal. However, I believe it helps. Tom Sabin introduced me to choline as a dietary supplement. After I started taking it, I felt as though my memory for names, and particularly the individual histories of patients, improved. This may be a placebo effect, and it may not reflect any direct change in the memory process but rather an improvement in my ability to concentrate and focus my attention so that new memories or engrams are encoded more efficiently.

In formulating our vitamin preparation, we specifically wanted to avoid including excessive levels of vitamins because, for example, too much pyridoxine (vitamin B-6) causes a disorder of the sensory part of the nervous system, especially in the ganglia situated alongside the spinal cord. We also did not include excitatory amino acids, like glutamic acid, in this formula either, since in normal circumstances a transport system in the blood-brain barrier moves excess glutamic acid away from brain cells. If the transport system fails because of a breakdown in the blood-brain barrier, too much glutamic acid will accumulate around brain cells, leading to a concentration of calcium ions and the death of brain cells.

I also recommend that you drink forty-five to sixty ounces of pure water a day, provided kidney and heart function are normal.* Of course, fruit juices or skimmed milk (for those who do not have lactose intolerance) can be substituted for water.

What about people with a family history of early heart disease or stroke? Such persons should reduce the total amount of fat in their diets, relying chiefly on fish, chicken, and turkey (without the skin) to supply protein. Deep-sea fish, such as salmon and tuna, are particularly good choices because of the essential fatty acids they contain. Most kinds

---

*I drink bottled water because tap water in many locations contains an excessive amount of chlorine, which may injure the bladder lining.

of high-fat meat should be avoided. Eggs — hard- or soft-boiled — have good nutritional value, even though they do contain cholesterol; one or two can be eaten once or twice a week. Avoid butter, margarine made with hydrogenated oil, peanut butter made with hydrogenated oil, ice cream, cream, whole milk, desserts made with lard or vegetable shortening, and foods fried in lard or shortening.

Because hypertension is often associated with early heart disease and stroke, a diet low in sodium should be initiated — which means not merely not adding table salt but also avoiding many canned foods and soups, which are loaded with sodium. Moreover, control the total number of calories taken in if weight is a problem. Olive oil and vinegar dressings with condiments such as garlic and onions added are preferable to commercial high-calorie salad dressings, and soybean desserts, such as diet Tofutti, taste like ice cream but have almost no fat and reduced calories. Also, although this item isn't strictly related to diet, people with heart disease or stroke in their families should avoid the use of tobacco.

Contrary to the usual practice of Americans, it is important that you eat your largest meal in the morning, including fish, chicken, or turkey; you can then snack during the day on low-fat foods like vegetables and fruits and have a very small amount to eat at night just before going to bed, when the calories taken in will not be used up immediately.

Another sure way to avoid weight gain is to buy a doctor's scale. Unlike inaccurate spring scales, shifting weight from one foot to another on a balance beam scale will not reduce your weight by five to eight pounds. If you are gaining weight or not losing it as you'd like, it means one thing: you have to cut down on your food intake. Losing extra pounds can be more difficult for some people than for others if they have a genetic predisposition to being overweight. Even so, the body is fundamentally a heat machine. To maintain constant weight, calories in must equal calories out. If we take in more

213

calories than we use up, we will store the excess as fat in our bodies. Generally speaking, people who weigh less are less prone to heart attacks and strokes than those who are overweight.

Exercise and Health

Will exercise help us avoid the kind of strokes associated with hardening of the arteries or arteriosclerotic disease? Yes, I believe it will, but that doesn't mean you have to be able to run a six-minute mile, or swim three hundred yards every morning, or go into a weight room for a forty-five-minute daily workout. As we get older our joints are more susceptible to injury from vigorous exercise, so I suggest any of the following programs to be done on a daily basis:

- walking or bicycling for forty-five minutes a day (walking to be done at three to four miles an hour)
- swimming for twenty to thirty minutes a day
- gentle jogging for twelve to fifteen minutes a day
- gentle resistance exercises and calisthenics for ten minutes a day

Keeping the body musculature toned up with calisthenic exercises is important. It's especially helpful to do sit-ups with the knees bent so that the abdominal muscles remain firm and strong and no undue strain is put on the back muscles. If one then has an occasional accidental fall, the body posture can be maintained by strong abdominal muscles aiding the back muscles in protecting against serious back and head injury.

Less demanding aerobic exercises like walking have to be done for a longer period of time than, say, running to get the same effect. But unlike some experts, who are satisfied with seeing people exercise three times a week, I believe in exercising daily — but I run only a mile and a half, not five miles.

214

Brain Exercises

Are there any specific brain exercises that can be done to help you improve or retain memory? Yes, and they are of several kinds. The first are preventive to make sure that as much brain function is retained after brain injuries or strokes as possible, and to aid in the rehabilitation process. Examples of these exercises are learning to write, or at least print, with the nondominant hand (usually the left); learning to get visual cues from the left visual field; and shaving or brushing one's teeth with the nondominant hand. Of course, such learning is much more effective if it's done before the age of five. But even in old age it has some protective effect if it is done before a stroke or injury.

Practicing all aspects of intellectual function and improving them as much as possible, although they aren't absolute preventives as far as Alzheimer's disease is concerned, certainly help to slow down the brain's aging process in the normal individual. Math skills should be practiced, including balancing your checkbook without a calculator, drawing with either hand, reading, and particularly reading aloud should also be a part of your mental practice.

More specific exercises to hone memory skills should focus on attention, concentration, and avoiding distraction. (Ideally, such skills should be practiced from kindergarten on, but it's never too late to begin. A complete program of these exercises can be found in my previous book, *Brain Power*.) In exercises to improve attention, an individual estimates the amount of time that has gone by and is checked by an observer with a stopwatch, concentrating enough to estimate intervals of ten seconds, twenty seconds, sixty seconds.

In another set of exercises, an examiner shows the subject various letters of the alphabet and associates each with a number. The subject is given time to memorize the letters and their corresponding numbers, which represent increments of time. The examiner then holds up a letter and instructs the subject to stop a watch when the elapsed time equals the numerical value of the letter.

A number of memory exercises, though they have not been effective in rehabilitating brain-injured people, do help expand the memory functions of normal individuals. These exercises enhance the ability to retain certain memories, and anyone can potentially profit from their use. Based on the association method of memory (sometimes called mnemonics), they involve correlating items to be remembered with other known information. Using these techniques, however, is like learning French or algebra: it requires time and concentration. The several varieties of mnemonics do work, sometimes in a spectacular fashion, but you must keep practicing them. Once you discover a memory technique that works for you, incorporate it into a short daily exercise routine.

Besides physical and mental exercises, your routine should include brain relaxation exercises. Relaxation doesn't mean allowing yourself to crumble into a heap and allow whatever unwarranted or unwanted thoughts that are on the scene parade through your mind. It means excluding everything that's going on in your environment, usually by sitting in a darkened room in a semireclining position with your eyes closed and a minimum of noise around you, and practicing a concentration technique to focus your attention.

Many different methods of relaxation are available, including autohypnosis, which is part of the conditioned reflex program defined by psychologist Andrew Salter; the "relaxation response" to induce lower blood pressure, written about by Herbert Benson; the system of Transcendental Meditation; and a number of other similar techniques.

One method I have advocated for achieving brain relaxation takes advantage of the physiological fact that certain portions of the anatomy, particularly the lips, tongue, index fingers, and great toes, are better represented on the surface of the brain (the cortex) than are other anatomical structures. To try this technique, eliminate all distractions and sit quietly with your eyes closed in the relaxation position. Focus your attention on relaxing the tip of your right thumb and work backward to the first joint, then the second. Concentrate on the anatomical structure of your thumb. After thirty to sixty seconds have passed, repeat the exercise, this time focusing on the middle and little fingers of your right hand. When you're finished with your right hand you can begin on your left; then on the right part of your tongue, the tip of the tongue, and the left part of the tongue; then on the muscles around your lips. Proceed to the eyelids on the right, first the upper, then the lower, and then transfer to the left side. If you're not completely relaxed at this time, go to the toes on your feet, beginning with the great toe on your right side.

Don't start these relaxation exercises when you're tense or upset; doing so will cause you to form bad conditioned reflexes, and the relaxation will not work. Rather, practice them first when you are relaxed so you can develop strong conditioned reflexes, which can eventually be applied in stressful situations. In my opinion relaxation exercises should be interspersed with memory exercises to achieve the best results. I also suggest that they be done in conjunction with physical exercises and mental exercises involving other parts of the brain, such as drawing, reading, and calculating.

Finally, to maintain brain fitness it is important to focus your attention on other people and other things. In any case, do not focus your attention on yourself. The more you think of yourself — your pleasures, what's in it for you — the more apt you are to become bored, fatigued, and ultimately depressed, with the kind of depression accompanied by hypochondriasis, easy distractibility, and loss of memory. This is the lesson taught by Mother Teresa, Dr. Albert Schweitzer, and St. Francis of Assisi. Never give up your interest in other people and other things. Always accept outside challenges as long as they are matched by your own talents and enthusiasm.

Vital Memory Points to Remember
1. Using appropriate brain exercises to keep your brain challenged and active will help maintain brain health.
2. The best way to reduce the risk of brain injury and memory loss is through having air bags installed and using three-point safety belts in automobiles.
3. Avoiding brain poisons of all kinds will greatly reduce your chance of suffering memory loss.
4. Dietary supplements, particularly of certain B vitamins, can help people who are concerned about memory loss from malnutrition.

20

Predictions: Preventing and Reversing Memory Loss

Alzheimer's Disease

WE WILL HAVE effective treatments for some forms of Alzheimer's disease in the next twenty years.* I believe that many of the necessary technical tools will be available in ten years, but population testing and government regulations may extend the time required to make these treatments available to all patients.

Alzheimer's is the most frequent irreversible cause of memory loss in the elderly, and its effective treatment will depend on early and accurate diagnosis, which, I predict, will take place in three years.

Beta amyloid protein, a complex of forty-two amino acids, is associated with brain cell death in Alzheimer's disease. This protein is present beneath the skin in Alzheimer's patients, and an abnormal amyloid protein, A-68, is found in patients' spinal fluid. I believe that either a spinal fluid examination or a skin biopsy will be the method used to confirm the diagnosis of Alzheimer's. Perhaps a monoclonal antibody will be used as a detector.

---

*The predictions in this chapter are based on the assumption that sufficient financial support will be available to carry out the necessary research.

219

The memory loss in Alzheimer's disease is correlated with a reduction in levels of the neurotransmitter acetylcholine in areas of the brain where new memories are formed. New drugs are now being introduced to increase the amount of acetylcholine in the brain. One of these, Tacrine, helped 40 percent of the members of one group of Alzheimer's patients. The drug may be toxic to the liver, however, and some researchers were not able to give sufficient amounts of the agent to get a therapeutic effect.

I predict that newer drugs to enhance acetylcholine effects will be available in four years. Some of these will very slowly and constantly release substances similar to acetylcholine into the spinal fluid. Others will enhance brain metabolism and improve memory by activating acetylcholine mechanisms within the brain itself.

I also predict that we will develop chemicals that will promote the survival and growth of nerve cells. One of these may be a genetically engineered nerve cell growth factor. Furthermore, I predict that within ten years we will be able to transplant fetal brain cells into the brains of Alzheimer's patients to replace their dead or dying cells. I believe that we will be able to harvest and grow such cells in brain cell cultures located in cell banks across the country. Through advances in genetic engineering, these cells will be transplanted into the host without the need for immunosuppressant drugs to inactivate the body's immune system so the cells will not be rejected.

New drugs will be developed to keep brain cells from being destroyed. Drugs already in use prevent brain cell death from excess calcium ions, but I predict that within the next five years drugs that inhibit the enzyme activity essential for the buildup of beta amyloid, the compound that may be responsible for nerve cell death in Alzheimer's, will be available.

Researchers will find more than one gene connected to

Alzheimer's disease, and on the basis of genetic classification alone we will find that what we now know as Alzheimer's disease actually comprises at least three different diseases, each with a different cause and treatment.

Multi-Infarct Dementia (Small Strokes)

I predict that we will reduce the incidence and severity of multi-infarct dementia, the second leading cause of irreversible memory loss in the elderly, in the next eight years. We will develop noninvasive tests to determine who is at risk for the disease, and we will develop new antihypertensive medications that will carry a smaller risk of low blood pressure in the blood vessels of the brain than that posed by the agents now in use.

We will have emergency techniques to unplug occluded blood vessels in the brain while they are in the process of producing an acute stroke. Such a technique might be to immediately insert a catheter into the blocked blood vessels and squirt in a clot-dissolving liquid, or to insert a fiberoptic scope into the blood vessel and pulverize the clot with either a new kind of laser or focused ultrasound, neither of which will damage the blood vessel wall.

New medications will be developed to reverse the arteriosclerotic process that results in narrowing of blood vessels. I believe this will be a boon to many Americans, who won't have gone on low-fat diets, even though high-fat diets endanger their health.

Within the next twenty years, genetic engineering will enable doctors to change the genetic makeup of those of us whose genes make us susceptible to early heart attack and stroke. Without restricting our diets, we will be able to maintain clean, healthy arteries and live vigorously into advanced old age.

221

The Brain as an Electrochemical System

Within the next twenty years you're going to see many people walking around with electrodes strapped to their scalps. They will look as though they have tape players piping music into their ears, but it won't be music playing. Instead, electrodes will deliver electrical or electromagnetic currents to their heads. These tiny currents will increase the level of certain neurotransmitters in the spinal fluid, such as serotonin, and will not only reverse depression but also correct associated memory problems.

These electrodes will reduce the amount of prescription tranquilizers and street drugs consumed by people. It should also entirely eliminate the need for drugs that have toxic effects on the brain. I do not advocate that people who aren't ill use transcranial electrical brain stimulation. But once people understand that their brains are electrochemical mechanisms that can be influenced by electrical current as well as by chemicals or drugs, it may be impossible to stop the widespread use of such devices to promote a feeling of relaxation.

Very weak transcranial electrical stimulation was first experimented with in the late fifties. Soviet doctors used it as an anesthetic, and in this country two psychiatrists reversed depression in severely depressed patients resistant to medication.

In 1965, Frank Ervin, Sol Aranow, and I applied very weak direct currents to the scalps of depressed patients. The currents had no effect in about a third of the patients, a transient beneficial effect in another third, and profound effects in reversing depression in the last third. These weak electrical currents produced changes in the brain's electromagnetic field, which in turn generated a current that stimulated the limbic portions of the brain. In patients who had a striking improvement in their depression, we found that the direction of flow of the direct current was important in producing the

222

beneficial effect. Reversing the direction of flow reversed the effect on the patients' depression.

An inventor and electrical engineer, Mr. Sol Liss, observing some of the work going on in our laboratory, altered an electronic device he had invented for transcutaneous electrical stimulation of nerves to relieve pain. In effect, he invented a new kind of cranial-stimulating device which supplied current in tiny amounts (he determined that the brain is most responsive to current alternating at fifteen cycles a second), one that effectively produced the changes in mood we were seeking.

In the last fifteen years, he and a number of clinical groups cooperating with him in the United States and Europe have applied this kind of current to the brains of about fifty thousand patients, mostly for the treatment of pain but also for depression, spasticity, and drug addiction. Fewer than forty of these patients had any difficulty from the treatment, and most of these complaints were about skin irritation at the site of the stimulation. None of the complaints was serious — a remarkable result that is in marked contrast to the adverse effects brought about by any medication to change brain function. Antidepressants, antipsychotics, sedatives, tranquilizers — almost every one has some toxic effect on the brain and brain function, and the percentage of patients taking them who are adversely affected is substantial. In addition, many of the psychoactive drugs are potentially addictive. Transcranial electrical stimulation has shown no such potential, at least in the patients who have been treated over the last fifteen years.

One of the studies that Mr. Liss and his colleagues did was reported at the First International Conference on Stress in Montreaux, Switzerland, in December 1988. The lead investigator in this study was Dr. C. Norman Shealy, a physician from Springfield, Missouri, who completed his training in

223

neurosurgery at the Massachusetts General Hospital.

Dr. Shealy first performed the study on fourteen normal, nonsmoking adults with no known illnesses and who were taking no drugs. Serving as controls, they ranged in age from twenty-two to seventy-two. In addition, another group of fourteen patients who suffered chronic pain ranged in age from thirty to sixty-eight. A third group consisted of nine chronic pain patients who considered their cases hopeless and were unable or unwilling to enter any usual kind of therapy program.

The fourth and last group in the study was composed of eleven patients with long-standing depression that had lasted for more than two years. All of these patients had been tried on a number of antidepressants and were unresponsive to two or more of these drugs. In fact, antidepressant drug therapy was so unsuccessful that the patients had discontinued therapy at the time of the stimulation. The oldest member of the group was sixty-seven and the youngest thirty.

All patients participating in the study were given thorough evaluations of their medical history and physical condition, and numerous laboratory studies were made. They received twenty minutes of transtemporal, transcranial stimulation at between one-half and one milliamp of current, just enough to evoke a visual flicker as a result of the electrical stimulation. Blood studies were done before the stimulation to provide a base line and again ten minutes after stimulation.

In the fourteen normal individuals, no substantial change occurred in blood levels of neurotransmitters — namely, in levels of serotonin, beta endorphins, norepinephrine, and cholinesterase. The same was true of the twenty-three chronic pain patients. In the eleven severely depressed patients, however, serotonin levels in the blood dramatically increased while cholinesterase declined.

After two weeks of daily transcranial stimulation, 60 percent of the depressed patients had significantly improved in psychological evaluations on a test for depression, and 50 percent of these patients had indications that they were no longer suffering clinical depression. Moreover, five of the nine chronic pain patients who were treated only with transcranial stimulation improved 50 percent or more in their estimates of total pain.

Of course, the clinical results here are suggestive, but not decisive. Long-term randomized, double-blind studies must be carried out to assess statistically the benefits of transcranial electrical stimulation. I predict these benefits will be significant, and that the technique will also enhance the effectiveness of antidepressant medication in much lower dosages.

Recently I've been prescribing transcranial electrical brain stimulation for patients who have failed to find relief from standard therapies. One of them is Zina, a fifty-two-year-old woman who had suffered multiple injuries in an automobile crash. Two years of treatment by physical therapy and various medications produced no real relief either in the pain from her injured left brachial plexus (at the base of her neck), which radiated into her left arm, or in her depressed mood. After only one week of transcutaneous electrical nerve stimulation, combined with transcranial brain stimulation, done three times a day for a period of twenty minutes, Zina had only minimal improvement of the pain in her brachial plexus, but her mood change was remarkable. When I first saw her she was extremely depressed and felt that her situation was hopeless. She admitted that she was suicidal. After only one week of transcranial stimulation, she was encouraging me. She said, "Doctor, I feel as though I'm going to get better. I know I still have some pain, but it doesn't bother me as much as it did before. I'm going to keep on with this. I'm feeling better." Four weeks after that she was ebullient — almost euphoric — and said that the pain, which was still present, didn't bother her.

The Future of Transcranial Electrical Brain Stimulation

Evidence is mounting that transcranial electrical brain stimulation can decrease drug dependence in abusers of some drugs, including heroin, cocaine, alcohol, and even prescription drugs. I predict that this technique will be widely used in the treatment of drug dependency in the next five years.

Since this kind of electrical stimulation seems to relieve depression (often present in drug and alcohol abusers) as one of its primary modes of action, the loss of memory associated with depression, produced by hyperdistractibility — the inability to concentrate or focus attention — should be relieved. Especially in persons over forty-five who have mild depression and complain of memory loss, transcranial stimulation may be of significant value. I predict that in the next five to ten years transcranial electrical brain stimulation will become an important treatment for depression and its associated memory loss.

Dr. Allan Chiles of Austin, Texas, who directs a rehabilitation hospital for the severely brain-injured, has recently reported that transcranial electrical stimulation has helped to reduce the memory loss of several patients with persistent post-traumatic amnesia. I predict that within the next five years transcranial electrical stimulation will help rouse stuporous, brain-injured patients into consciousness.

Finally, I predict that new discoveries about the frequencies and intensities of electrical currents and electromagnetic fields will allow them to be focused on the head in such a way as to selectively stimulate both deep and superficial areas of the brain in the treatment of a number of psychiatric and neurobehavioral symptoms. I predict that transcranial electrical brain stimulation will become widely used by physicians in psychiatry and rehabilitation medicine.

Conclusions and Summary

1. Loss of vital memory isn't part of normal aging.
2. True loss of vital memory means that you have a physical problem and need medical assessment.
3. A memory problem can best be defined by memory testing and a neurological examination.
4. Early diagnosis and prompt treatment can completely reverse many memory problems while making others less severe and more manageable.
5. There are methods to help you avoid memory problems and make your memory more efficient.
6. It is hoped that in a few years even the most severe memory problems will be treatable and, in another decade, preventable.

Bibliography

Scholarly Books and Articles

Adams, R. D., and M. Victor. *Principles of Neurology*. 3rd ed. New York: McGraw-Hill, 1985.

Alvarez-Buylla, A., J. Kirn, and F. Nottebohm. "Birth of Projection Neurons in Adult Avian Brain May Be Related to Perceptual or Motor Learning." *Science* 249 (1990):1444–46.

Barnes, H. N., M. D. Aronson, and T. L. Delbanco, eds. *Alcoholism: A Guide for the Primary Care Physician*. New York: Springer-Verlag, 1987.

Beaton, G. H., and J. M. Bengoa, eds. *Nutrition in Preventive Medicine*. Geneva: World Health Organization, 1976.

Beatty, W. W. "Opiate Antagonists, Morphine and Spatial Memory in Rats." *Pharmacology, Biochemistry and Behavior* 19 (1983):397–401.

Blaney, P. H. "Affect and Memory: A Review." *Psychological Bulletin* 99 (1986):229–46.

Block, R. I., and J. R. Wittenborn. "Marijuana Effects on the Speed of Memory Retrieval in the Letter-matching Task." *International Journal of the Addictions* 21 (1986):281–85.

———. "Marijuana Effects on Semantic Memory." *Psychological Reports* 55 (1984):503–512.

Bolla, K., et al. "Memory Complaints in Older Adults." *Archives of Neurology* 48 (1991):61–64.

229

Bibliography

Butters, N., and L. Cermak. *Alcoholic Korsakoff's Syndrome.* New York: Academic Press, 1980.

Church, A. C., et al. "Long-Term Suppression of the Cerebral Spread of a Memory: Effects of Idazoxan and Clonidine." *Pharmacology, Biochemistry and Behavior* 32 (1989):749–56.

Croog, S., et al. "The Effects of Antihypertensive Therapy on the Quality of Life." *New England Journal of Medicine* 314 (1986): 1657–64.

Davidoff, D. A., H. R. Kessler, D. F. Laibstain, and V. H. Mark. "Neurobehavioral Sequelae of Minor Head Injury: A Consideration of Post-Concussive Syndrome Versus Past Traumatic Stress Disorder." *Cognitive Rehabilitation* (March/April 1988): 8–13.

Ellis, H. C. "On the Importance of Mood Intensity and Encoding Demands in Memory: Commentary on Hasher, Rose, Zacks, Sanft, and Doren." *Journal of Experimental Psychology* 114 (1985): 392–95.

Ervin, F. R., S. Aranow, and V. H. Mark. "Low Level DC Polarization in Man: Clinical Behavioral and Electrophysiologic Observations." *Abstracts of the Conference on Effects of Diffuse Electrical Currents on Physiological Mechanisms with Application to Electroanesthesia and Electrosleep* 4 (1966):23.

Fitten, L., et al. "Treatment of Alzheimer's Disease with Short- and Long-Term Oral THA and Lecithin." *American Journal of Psychiatry* 147 (1990):239–42.

Fossen, A., et al. "Effects of Hypnotics on Memory." *Pharmacology* 27, supp. 2 (1983):116–26.

Fulginiti, S., and L. Cancela. "Effect of Naloxone and Amphetamine on Acquisition and Memory Consolidation of Active Avoidance Responses in Rats." *Psychopharmacology* 79 (1983):45–48.

Gawin, F. H., and E. H. Ellingwood. "Cocaine and Other Stimulants." *New England Journal of Medicine* 318 (1988):1173–82.

Greenwood, C. "The Role of Diet in Modulating Brain Metabolism and Behavior." *Contemporary Nutrition* 14, no. 7 (1989).

Griffith, H. W. *Complete Guide to Vitamins, Minerals, and Supplements.* Tucson: Fisher, 1988.

Hall, S., and R. Bornstein. "The Relationship Between Intelligence and Memory Following Minor or Mild Closed Head Injury." *Journal of Neurosurgery* 75 (1991):378–81.

Harrell, R. F. "Mental Response to Added Thiamine." *Journal of Nutrition* 31 (1946):283–98.

Hartley, L. R., et al. "The Effect of Beta Adrenergic Blocking Drugs on Speakers' Performance and Memory." *British Journal of Psychiatry* 142 (1983):512–17.

Hilton, H. *The Executive Memory Guide.* New York: Simon and Schuster, 1986.

Horn, J. L. "Psychometric Studies of Aging and Intelligence." In *Aging: Genesis and Treatment of Psychological Disorders in the Elderly,* edited by Gersons and Rankin, 19–43. New York: Raven Press, 1975.

Izquierdo, I., and M. Graudenz. "Memory Facilitation by Naloxone Is Due to Release of Dopaminergic and Beta-Adrenergic Systems from Tonic Inhibition." *Psychopharmacology* 67 (1980):265–68.

Katzman, R., and R. D. Terry, eds. *The Neurology of Aging.* Philadelphia: Davis, 1984.

Kirk, A., and A. Kertesz. "On Drawing Impairment in Alzheimer's Disease." *Archives of Neurology* 48 (1991):73–77.

Kirk, R. C., K. White, and N. McNaughton. "Low Dose Scopolamine Affects Discriminability but Not Rate of Forgetting in Delayed Conditional Discrimination." *Psychopharmacology* 96 (1988):541–46.

Lee, J. C. "The Effects of Alcohol Injections on the Blood-Brain Barrier." *Quarterly Journal of Studies on Alcohol* 23 (1962):4–16.

Loke, Wing H. "Effects of Caffeine on Mood and Memory." *Physiology and Behavior* 44 (1988):367–72.

Madrazo, L. V., et al. "Transplantation of Fetal Substantia Nigra and Adrenal Medulla to the Caudate Nucleus in Two Patients with Parkinson's Disease." *New England Journal of Medicine* 318 (1988):51.

Mark, V. H., et al. "The Destruction of Both Anterior Thalamic Nuclei in a Patient with Intractable Agitated Depression." *Journal of Nervous and Mental Disease* 150 (1970): 266–72.

231

Bibliography

Mark, V. H., and F. R. Ervin. *Violence and the Brain*. New York: Harper and Row, 1970.

Mark, V. H., F. Ervin, and W. Sweet. "Deep Temporal Lobe Stimulation in Man." In *The Neurobiology of the Amygdala*, edited by Basil E. Eleftheriou, 485–507. New York: Plenum, 1971.

Mark, V. H., with J. P. Mark. *Brain Power*. Boston: Houghton Mifflin, 1989.

McGlone, J., et al. "Screening for Early Dementia Using Memory Complaints from Patients and Relatives." *Archives of Neurology* 47 (1990):1189–93.

Meier, M. J., A. Benton, and L. Diller, eds. *Neuropsychological Rehabilitation*. New York: Guilford, 1987.

Mesulam, M.-M., ed. *Principles of Behavioral Neurology*. Philadelphia: Davis, 1988.

Miyamoto, M., et al. "Effects of Continuous Infusion of Cholinergic Drugs on Memory Impairment in Rats with Basal Forebrain Lesions." *Journal of Pharmacology and Experimental Therapeutics* 248 (1989):825–35.

Moore, R. G., F. N. Watts, and J. Williams. "The Specificity of Personal Memories in Depression." *British Journal of Clinical Psychology* 27 (1988):275–76.

Moskowitz, H., and M. Burns. "The Effects on Performance of Two Antidepressants, Alone and in Combination with Diazepam." *Progress in Neuro-Psychopharmacological and Biological Psychiatry* 12 (1988):783–92.

Nolan, K. A., et al. "A Trial of Thiamine in Alzheimer's Disease." *Archives of Neurology* 48 (1991):81–83.

Norton, N. A., et al. "Memory for Event Frequency as a Function of Depression, Age, Intentionality, and Level of Processing." *Journal of General Psychology* 115 (1988):369–81.

Quartermain, D., M. Judge, and H. Jung. "Amphetamine Enhances Retrieval Following Diverse Sources of Forgetting." *Physiology and Behavior* 43 (1988):239–41.

Richardson, P. J., and M. A. Wyke. "Memory Function: Effects of Different Antihypertensive Drugs." *Drugs* 35, supp. 5 (1988): 80–85.

Sabin, T. D. "Dementia in the Elderly: Identifying Reversibility." *Hospital Practise*, November 30, 1986.

Sabin, T. D., and V. H. Mark, eds. "Boston City Hospital Ground Rounds: A Case of Intractable Rage." *Behavioral Medicine* (July 1981):32–41.

Sabin, T. D., A. J. Vitug, and V. H. Mark. "Are Nursing Home Diagnoses and Treatment Inadequate?" *Journal of the American Medical Association* 248 (1982):321–22.

Salem, S. A., and D. G. McDevitt. "Central Effects of Beta-Adreno-ceptor Antagonists." *Clinical Pharmacology and Therapeutics* (1983):52–57.

Salzman, C. *Clinical Geriatric Psychopharmacology*. New York: Mc-Graw-Hill, 1984.

Sass, K., et al. "The Neural Substrate of Memory Impairment Demonstrated by the Intracarotid Amobarbital Procedure." *Archives of Neurology* 48 (1991):48–52.

Shealy, C., et al. "Depression: A Diagnostic, Neurochemical Profile and Therapy with Cranial Electrical Stimulation (CES)." *Journal of Neurological and Orthopaedic Medicine and Surgery* 10 (December 1989).

———. "Therapy with Cranial Electrical Stimulation (CES)." Paper presented at the First International Conference on Stress. Montreaux, Switzerland, December 1988.

Squire, L., and N. Butters. *Neuropsychology of Memory*. New York: Guilford, 1984.

Stevens, J., et al. "Deep Temporal Stimulation in Man." *Archives of Neurology* 21 (1969):157–69.

Strub, R. L., and F. W. Black. *The Mental Status Examination in Neurology*. 2nd ed. Philadelphia: Davis, 1987.

Teasdale, J. D., and S. J. Fogarty. "Differential Effects of Induced Mood on Retrieval of Pleasant and Unpleasant Events from Episodic Memory." *Journal of Abnormal Psychology* 88 (1979):248–57.

Turney, M. C., et al. "The NINCPS-ARDRA Work Group Criteria for the Clinical Diagnosis of Probable Alzheimer Disease." *Neurology* 38 (1988):359.

Venna, N., et al. "Reversible Depression in Binswanger's Disease." *Journal of Clinical Psychiatry* 49 (January 1988):23–26.

Victor, M., R. Adams, and G. Collins. *The Wernicke-Korsakoff Syndrome*. Philadelphia: Davis, 1989.

Vyse, S. A., and M. D. Rapport. "The Effects of Methylphenidtae on Learning in Children with ADDH." *Journal of Consulting and Clinical Psychology* 57 (1989):425–35.

Wurtman, R. J., et al., eds. *Alzheimer's Disease.* Proceedings of the Fifth Meeting of the International Study Group on the Pharmacology of Memory Disorders Associated with Aging. Zurich, Switzerland, January 20–22, 1989.

Newspaper Articles

Angier, Natalie. "Gains Seen in Diagnostic Test for Alzheimer's." *New York Times,* June 6, 1990, p. A24.

Blakeslee, Sandra. "The Brain May 'See' What Eyes Cannot." *New York Times,* January 15, 1991, p. C1.

Eckholm, Erik. "Haunting Issue for U.S.: Caring for the Elderly Ill." *New York Times,* March 27, 1990, p. A1.

Kolata, Gina. "Gene Mutation That Causes Alzheimer's Is Found." *New York Times,* February 16, 1991, p. A1.

———. "The Aging Brain: The Mind Is Resilient, It's the Body That Fails." *New York Times,* April 16, 1991, p. C1.

Lewin, Tamar. "Strategies to Let Elderly Keep Some Control." *New York Times,* March 28, 1990, p. A1.

Lublin, Joann S. "Alzheimer's Linked to Aluminum in Water." *Wall Street Journal,* January 13, 1988, p. B2.

Martin, Douglas. "How to Preserve a Strong Mind: Flex It Regularly." *New York Times,* March 10, 1990, p. A27.

Waldholz, Michael. "Iron-Reducing Drug Is Found to Slow the Effects of Alzheimer's, Study Says." *Wall Street Journal,* May 31, 1991, p. B4.

Index

Index

Alzheimer's disease (*cont.*)
  treatment of, 37, 140, 193, 194,
    197–98, 199, 219–221
  verbal abilities and, 18
  vital memory loss and, 18, 39
Amino acids, 123
Amnesia, post-traumatic, 226
Amphetamines, 39, 52, 75, 76, 78,
  208
Anemia, 107, 108, 109, 127, 128,
  129–31, 156–57
Angel Dust, 39, 82, 208
Angiotensin-converting enzyme
  inhibitors, 92
Antibiotics, 111, 141, 145, 146, 150,
  151
Antidepressants, 50, 57, 59–61, 89–
  91, 95, 173, 223, 224
Antiemetics, 93–94
Antihypertensive drugs, 90–92,
  171, 172, 174, 175, 178, 208, 221
Antipsychotics, 223
Anxiety, 52, 53, 80, 172, 174–75.
  See also Panic disorders
Apathy, 107, 136, 186
Aranow, Sol, 222
Arsenic poisoning, 209
Arteriosclerosis, 127, 214, 221
Arteriovenous malformations, 164
Artistic abilities, 7, 18
Aspirin, 167
Asthma, 130
Atarax, 80
Atenolol, 91
Athletic abilities, 7, 19
Ativan, 53, 80, 208
Attention
  concentration, 15
  focus of, 13, 67
  lack of concentration, 54, 61, 64,
    226
  span, 12, 26, 61, 105
Automobile accidents, 152, 156–
  58, 159, 207
AZT, 149

Barbiturates, 39, 80, 87, 208
Behavioral neurology, 12, 15
Behavior modification, 7
Belladonna, 84, 85
Benson, Herbert, 216
Beriberi, 109
Beta amyloid protein, 219, 220
Beta blockers, 91, 175, 208
Binswanger's disease, 171–72, 173,
  188
Biopsy, brain, 141, 142
Biotin, 100
Blood
  acid-base balance, 116–18, 121,
    123
  -brain barrier, 66, 74, 208, 212
  calcium in, 133
  clots. *See* Subdural hematoma
  ketone bodies, 122, 123
  oxygen in, 98, 122, 127–31
  pressure (high and low), 165,
    171, 172–75, 177, 179, 213, 221
  sugar, 98, 122–27, 130–31, 136–
    37
  thinners, 167, 170
  transfusion, 204
  /urine testing, 42, 45, 118, 136,
    144, 146
  vessels and arteries, 165, 166,
    167, 168, 169, 221
Boston City Hospital, 101, 104, 164
Brain
  adrenal cortex, 133, 136
  auditory cortex, 8, 21
  cells, 86, 95, 119–20, 127, 130,
    212
  development, 7
  as electrochemical system, 222–
    25
  environmental cues to, 7–8, 12,
    15, 19–20
  frontal lobes, 21, 68, 71, 185–86
  hemorrhage, 164, 165, 166, 188
  hippocampus, 82, 94, 130, 131,
    144

236

Index

Computerized axial tomography. *See* CAT scans
Concentration. *See* Attention
Confabulation, 27, 28, 104
Copper, 196

Death of spouse or loved one, 33, 37, 50
Dehydration, 40, 98, 111, 112–13, 115, 121. *See also* Electrolytes
Dementia, 40, 41, 42, 135, 136
  brain disease and, 141, 142, 147, 149, 150
  depression misdiagnosed as, 50
  epilepsy and, 162
  memory loss and, 141
  multi-infarct, xi, 166–72, 178, 179, 204, 205
  See also Alzheimer's disease
Depressants, 80–81, 82–83
Depression, xi, 29, 30, 34, 37, 38, 194, 195, 196
  alcoholism and, 52–53, 64, 69
  brain disease and, 140, 149, 150
  brain injury and, 154, 155
  classifications, 50–51
  clinical, 51–53, 204, 225
  drug therapy for, 56, 57, 59, 60–61, 64
  in elderly, 41, 42, 46, 50, 58–61
  memory loss and, 49–50, 222, 226
  misdiagnosis of, 134, 150
  psychotherapy for, 50, 53, 57, 64
  reactive, 64
  severe, 56–61, 89
  street drugs and, 76, 78
  stress-related, 50, 53, 61–64
  stroke and, 170, 177, 178
  surgical therapy for, 57–58
  treatment of, 39, 56, 222, 223–25
Desyrel, 173
Diabetes, 92, 205, 208
Diabetes mellitus, 123–25
Diabetic coma, 116, 123, 124

Diet, 97–98, 221
  memory loss and, 209–14
  pills, 75, 76
Dietary supplements, 209–10, 218
Digitalis, 92, 208
Dilantin, 109, 164
Disability insurance, 155–56
Down's syndrome, 194
Drugs and drug abuse, 34, 39, 75, 222
  brain poisoning from, 75–76, 82–83, 140, 170, 195–96, 208
  depression and, 52–53, 76, 78
  designer, 81
  intravenous, 151
  stroke and, 170, 177
  See also Medication

Ear and sinus infection, 145–46, 151
Elavil, 89, 90, 208
Elderly
  brain and head injuries, 153, 154
  depression in, 41, 42, 46, 50, 58–61
  dietary supplements and, 102n, 108–9, 110
  drug therapy for, 81, 86
  electrolyte levels and, 114–15, 120
  epilepsy in, 162–63
  hydrocephalus and, 186–87, 188
  subdural hematomas in, 181–82
  vital memory testing in, 42–43
  See also Alzheimer's disease; Nursing homes
Electroencephalogram, 42, 45
Electrolytes, 98, 99, 120, 133
  brain and, 111–13, 140
  ions and, 113–15, 121
  low sodium syndrome and, 115
  See also Dehydration
Electroshock therapy, 56, 57, 61, 150
Emotions, 12, 13. *See also* Brain: limbic

Index

Index